MINDFUL
NEW MOM

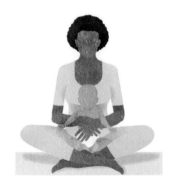

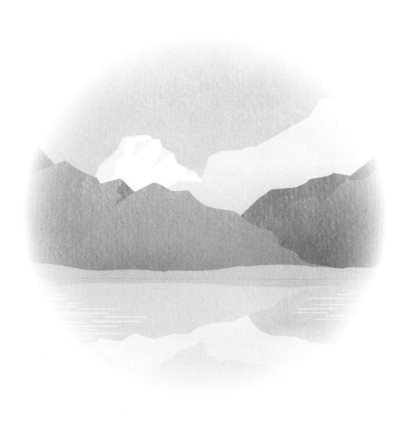

MINDFUL
NEW MOM

MEDITATION · YOGA · VISUALIZATION · NATURAL REMEDIES · NUTRITION
A MIND–BODY APPROACH TO THE HIGHS AND LOWS OF MOTHERHOOD

DR. CAROLINE BOYD

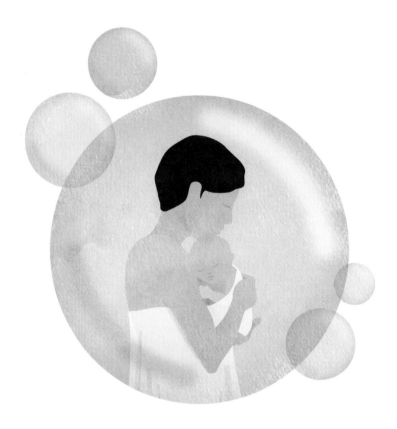

To my loves, Laurie,
Isla, and Reuben

Contents

Introduction

Becoming a mom is life-changing. Mindful compassion teaches you to open your heart to the highs and lows of mothering—enhancing everyday connections with yourself, your baby, and the world around you.

When I first became a mom, people told me, "Just trust your instincts." I remember thinking, "Okay, but how do I know what those instincts are?" Gradually, I understood that settling into my new role was a process, as I learned my baby's unique cues and what kind of mom I wanted to be. The idea that women are born knowing innately how to mother is a fairy tale, belonging to the Supermom myth. This has us believe we must always be coping, in control, and loving our role. The idea of Supermom stems from the Western ideology of motherhood in a patriarchal system, a central theme of this book. Much research cited is based broadly on Caucasian, educated groups—we need more diversity, amplifying more voices. I draw on some non-Western postpartum practices yet recognize these have constraints, too.

The messy reality of motherhood teaches us that living up to Supermom is impossible. In my experience working clinically with families adjusting to parenthood, many women (and men) struggle, each in their own ways. My hope in writing this book is to help you feel seen and understood amid the kaleidoscope of emotions arising on this journey. When you have a baby, you can feel shaken up like a snow globe. Up into the air go your prebaby identities, emotions, and

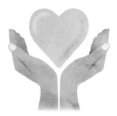

relationships. As you adjust, there is a unique opportunity for growth as you reevaluate old stories and patterns that no longer serve you.

Mindfulness allows you to shine a light on what's most helpful to you in any given moment. Instead of being bound up in your thoughts as "truths," adopting an "Observer" position gives you power to step back and respond with compassion. Living mindfully helps you turn down the noise and focus on what really matters. Identifying your parenting values empowers you to make choices that fit *your* family.

Parenting will inspire and test you. My take-home message for moms is that it's essential to look after yourself. As girls, we're often not taught to attend to our own needs, yet doing so is vital for our well-being. Use the meditations, affirmations, visualizations, yoga, nutritional advice, and natural remedies that feel right for you—nothing is prescriptive. I've integrated ideas from my clinical practice, research, and experience as a parent. Staying curious and reflective is key to mothering. It's okay *not* to know all the answers. I hope this book encourages you to develop a kinder relationship with yourself, helping you find more head and heart space to become the mom *you* want to be.

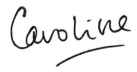

MINDFUL PARENTING

The transition to motherhood is tender and transformative. However, pressure to parent perfectly can make this adjustment difficult. Practicing mindful compassion provides tools to ground you during this time—allowing you to find calm, soothe your baby, and embrace being a new mom.

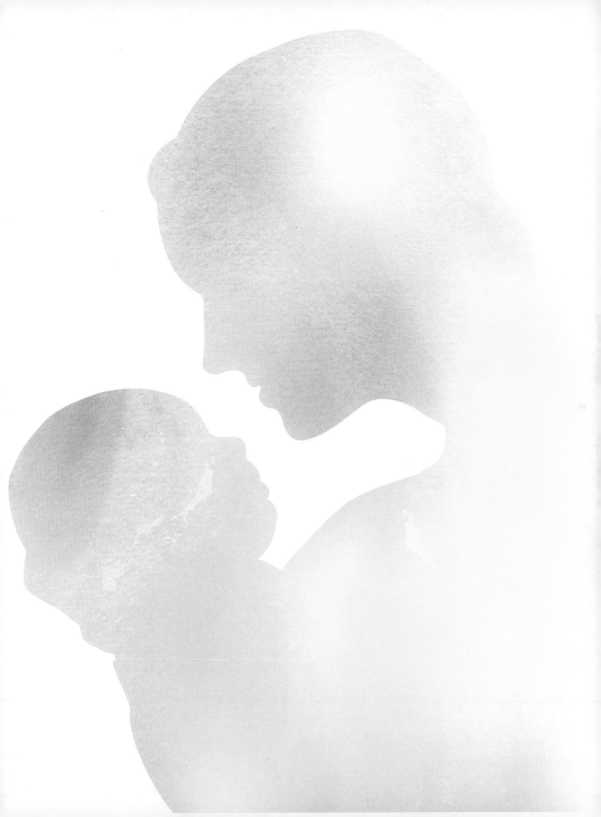

Being a Mindful Mother

Mindfulness is simply choosing to pay attention to the present moment, without judgment, whether you're feeding peacefully or soothing your baby. It allows you to open your heart to the highs and lows of parenting.

Perhaps you have already experienced that moment when you find yourself alone for the first time with your new baby. You may have wondered: "How have I been left in charge? Am I up to the job?" Parenting is one of the most challenging tasks you'll ever do, yet there's no manual. It's messy, a marvel, a muddling through. Mindful parenting allows you to connect with your rich inner experience and be more fully present with your baby—in the moment as it unfolds. Practicing mindfulness allows you to find ways to ground yourself and stand, steady as an oak tree, while the storms of parenting blow around you.

No doubt your child will bring you moments of tenderness, wonder, and joy, as well as triggering strong feelings and testing your limits. Instead of adding yet another pressure, mindfulness helps you tune in to the full range of feelings. Becoming more mindful allows you to notice difficult feelings as they arise rather than judge yourself for having them.

The roots of mindfulness lie in teachings of the Buddha, described by the Sanskrit word "dharma"—meaning "the way things are." Cultivating awareness means focusing attention inward to your thoughts, emotions, and bodily sensations—without resisting them or getting caught up in past worries or future fears.

Early motherhood can be stressful: acknowledging and accepting what is, including any difficult emotions, creates space to step back, allowing you to respond, not react. To let go of believing there's a "right" way to parent and that you "should" be doing things a certain way. To make wise choices for you and your baby, asking yourself in times of challenge: "What's most important here?"

Adopting a mindful approach

Using the six pillars of mindfulness (*see p13*) will help you flourish in your new role as a mother as you appreciate the values of patience, acceptance, trust, and letting go. You are likely to hold preconceived beliefs and hopes about becoming a mom, shaped by society and your own experiences. Perhaps you have a fantasy in your mind about how you will parent and how your baby will behave. You may feel crushed by expectations to parent perfectly. This is linked to the myth of "Supermom," which has us believe moms should always be calm, coping, and in control. Acknowledging when you may be striving to be Supermom creates space to respond wisely, without feeling the need to control.

It can also be hard to keep up with the constant changes: some days you may feel you're doing well, you're coping, you're winning. On other days, you may feel so tired and full of self-doubt—if only you could just get

>>

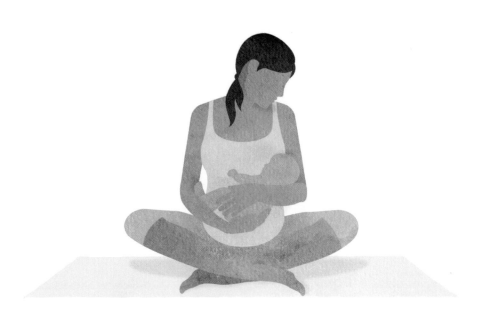

"Mindful mothering allows you to turn down all the noise and tune in to yourself and your baby."

it "right." Self-critical thoughts often arise amid stress, as you negatively label your present-moment experience. So if you feel bad, you then judge yourself for even feeling that way. Learning to redirect your attention allows you to step back from external pressures and quiet the mental chatter of your inner critic, easing doubts and fears.

Amid all the "doing" of mothering, mindfulness brings a unique opportunity to slow the pace of life, as you shift into "being" mode. Becoming more deeply connected to yourself, and in turn your baby, brings a kind of "heartfulness." Even on the most sleep-deprived days, these tools will help you find an anchor as you access calm within. The visualizations and values exercises will further support you to tap in to your own inner wisdom and become the mother *you* want to be.

Benefits of mindfulness

Research into mindful parenting is promising, highlighting many benefits. Practicing mindful parenting has been found to reduce parenting stress, with parents reporting better relationships with their children. Mindfulness group training for mothers and their babies has been linked to greater well-being, self-compassion, and confidence. By increasing mindful awareness, mothers were helped with how to cope with stress and to respond to their own needs as well as those of their babies.

Research also shows that mindful parenting can even change areas in the maternal brain. Mindful meditation can strengthen connections between our "thinking" brain (prefrontal cortex) responsible for planning and decision-making and our "emotional" brain (amygdala and brain stem).

SIX ATTITUDES OF MINDFULNESS

These interconnected "pillars" will support you to become a mindful mother as you attend to your thoughts and feelings, helping you become more connected to your baby.

Beginner's mind

You are likely to have preconceived ideas about being a mom. Cultivating beginner's mind means seeing each unique moment with a fresh pair of eyes—unclouded by expectations of motherhood and reactivity.

Nonjudging

Learning to recognize critical thoughts, including self-judging ones, helps you step back without getting hooked by them. Instead, notice thoughts with kindness as "mental events" flowing in and passing by like leaves in a stream.

Patience

It is said that patience is the highest form of love. Mindfulness teaches you to enhance your capacity for patience when you feel tested. Allowing your baby to find their own rhythm at their own pace requires both patience and compassion (*see p18*).

Trust

It's easy to feel overwhelmed by the volume of information both on- and offline. Developing trust in yourself as the expert of your own—and your baby's experience— allows you to tune in to your own intuition to make wise choices.

Acceptance

Acknowledging what is, including difficult emotions, can help you see the bigger picture. Instead of wishing things to be a certain way, this clarity moves you toward acceptance—opening up new possibilities.

Letting go

Mindfulness means letting go of impossible expectations, such as being Supermom, while bringing a kind curiosity to unpleasant feelings or situations. Let go of "should" and "must" around feeding and sleeping, allowing things to be as they are.

All About You

With the arrival of a baby comes the birth of a mother. This huge transition can come as a shock, both physically and emotionally. Mindfulness teaches you a new, kinder relationship with yourself.

You may feel acutely sensitive, raw, and vulnerable in this brand-new role you feel ill prepared for. You may feel full of pride along with disbelief and fear that you must learn on the job to care for this tiny human being. You may be powerfully in love with your baby yet feel trapped at home. You may welcome your new identity yet grieve losses from your prebaby life. These contradictory feelings are normal, as is the intense emotional upheaval of early motherhood.

Matrescence

It can be reassuring to understand the major shifts occurring in this transition in the context of "matrescence." This term, coined in 1973 by medical anthropologist Dana Raphael, was popularized by perinatal psychiatrist Dr. Alexandra Sacks. Matrescence compares the process of becoming a mother to the huge changes arising in adolescence. Just as teenagers navigate emotionally turbulent waters, so too do new moms through significant brain, body, and identity changes. Evidence suggests that women undergo shifts in the brain during pregnancy, lasting at least two years postpartum, that relate to heightened anxiety. Affected brain regions are associated with the ability

"Adjusting to your new identity takes time. Go gently."

to empathize and understand another's perspective. These changes are thought to prepare a mother to recognize her baby's needs, to respond to her baby sensitively, and to perceive threats. What this means is that feeling a strong desire to protect your baby and attend to their needs is understandable. You may at times feel overwhelmed by the sheer responsibility. These are signs that your amazing maternal brain is doing just what it's designed to do.

Adapting to your new role

Identity-wise, women often find the shift in tempo surprising. Perhaps you have an established career, in which you feel reasonably competent in your role. Adjusting to the slower pace of life at home with your baby, with all its hard-to-measure achievements, can take time. In a culture equating success with busyness and productivity, you may feel lost on those days lacking any predictability or order. What can compound a felt lack of control is the weight of external expectations. In part, this relates to the perfect mother myth, which places huge pressure on women to cope, maintain control, and be a "good" mom.

This powerful myth, internalized by women from an early age, has us believe we must be "Supermom, Superwife, Supereverything." It creates the idea that experiencing any negative feelings means you are bad or failing. Add to this major hormonal changes, broken sleep, and loss of community, and herein lies the perfect storm of modern motherhood. It's no wonder that one

in five women will experience a mood difficulty in the perinatal period. For advice on seeking help, see page 214.

Accepting support

What new mothers need is simply to feel held, heard, and understood. In the absence of society supporting the mother, what becomes crucial is the relationships that encircle us. Mindfully creating your Circle of Support (*see p78*) can identify trusted loved ones in your network and who is best placed to offer different kinds of support. Finding your tribe of like-minded female friends is part of this process.

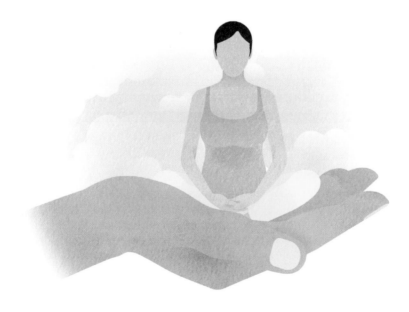

"Connecting with yourself in a mindful, compassionate way can be transformative."

Given that a new baby can place strain on the couple relationship, the partner exercises in this book will support you both to stay connected where possible.

At the center of your new family is the relationship between you and your baby, which will flourish and blossom over time as you get to know each other. Adopting a mindful approach to parenting will help you consciously shift from "doing" to "being" mode, as you learn ways to fall into step with your baby and find your rhythm together. Learning ways to contain your baby requires trial and error—and oodles of patience and empathy (*see p68*).

Cultivating mindful awareness

To offer a safe haven for your baby, you need to develop an internal place of safety as well as reach out to others to sustain you. After the birth, it can be harder to rely on your usual ways of coping to feel centered and grounded. Sleep and time for yourself is compromised along with doing activities you enjoy. A further layer of difficulty comes from feeling shame and berating yourself for even feeling certain emotions. This is why it is so important to bring understanding and compassion to *all* your feelings.

Practicing mindfulness teaches you to have a more accepting relationship with yourself—perhaps the hardest task of all in parenting. Learning to understand and acknowledge your feelings—love, fear, anger, sorrow—allows you to create space to respond wisely and teaches you that your emotions, however unpleasant, are always in flow and will pass. Getting to know your rich inner world also helps you become less governed by expectations and more in touch with yourself as a "good enough" mother (*see p113*).

A Compassionate Approach to Motherhood

Love, including mother-love, is multifaceted and ever-changing, evolving over time in response to continued compassion, effort, and care. For many women, mother-love grows as they become more confident in their role.

What does the powerful phrase "mother-love" mean to you? The love between a mom and baby induces hormonal surges similar to romantic love. Moments of connection release oxytocin and dopamine, producing feelings of warmth and elation. Yet dreamy euphoria is not the whole story.

Our ability to learn and grow as a mother depends on how nourished, safe, and supported we feel in our environment. In Western, individualistic cultures, isolation can create stress for women, who often shoulder the burden of mothering alone.

Another pressure facing modern moms is the idea that mothering is instinctive—we'll know innately what to do. The hopes, fantasies, and fears we bring to our new role are shaped by our own experiences of being parented, as well as by Supermom (*see p111*). So here we are, in this new chaos, expecting we ought to know but feeling a cocktail of emotions that don't fit society's joyful norm. These expectations can set us up to fail, increasing the pressure of motherhood. In reality, we learn on the job.

Self-care

So how best to navigate the challenges? Feeling supported by those around us is vital—yet it's the relationship with ourself that needs the most care and attention. The airplane oxygen mask analogy is helpful here—just as a mother needs to apply her own mask first, she must also learn to soothe herself before she can soothe her baby. Mindfulness teaches us to pay attention to our mind and body with compassion.

How the brain works

A first step in understanding why we can struggle with our emotions is learning about our "tricky" emotional brain. As human beings, we have two different brain systems—one of which functions similarly to animals' brains. This is our "emotional" brain, which evolved many millions of years ago and is highly sensitized to threat. It is hardwired for survival and reproduction, focused on keeping us and our newborn safe. Basic emotions such as fear, anger, and sadness direct defensive behaviors, triggering fight, flight, or freeze reactions.

What sets us apart from animals is our "thinking" brain. Located in our frontal lobes, this more recently evolved brain is responsible for using our attention, imagination, and ability to fantasize, think, reason, and plan. This higher consciousness and sense of self makes us human.

The problem is, the capacity to reflect on ourselves and how others perceive us can *create* suffering. For example, when our baby is unwell or we feel we've failed, our emotional brain hijacks our thinking brain. We get stuck in loops of anxiety and self-judgment.

»

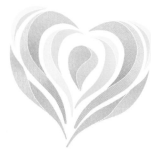

A compassionate approach

An antidote to suffering is compassion. Compassion is twofold: courage to turn toward suffering in ourselves and others—and taking responsibility to gently and firmly relieve that suffering.

Dealing with our "tricky" brain is part of our common humanity. This is a lifelong work of strengthening compassion through consciously connecting with it. Self-care isn't self-indulgent—it's about making compassionate choices, such as saying "no." Mindful compassion teaches us to notice emotions arising in mothering with kindness—helping us to tolerate them without self-blame.

Professor Paul Gilbert's adapted Three Circle model (right) shows the emotional systems helping us to survive and thrive.

Threat-focused system

Our threat system is shaped by our genes and life experiences. This system is highly sensitive and reactive. The stress of life with a new baby comes with many new anxieties, whether self-critical thoughts about not being good enough, fear of external judgment, or "What if" worries about our baby's safety. Just as a life-and-death threat, such as a predatory attack, triggers our internal alarm system, all these threats send the same "Danger!" signal—activating the fight, flight, freeze reaction in our sympathetic nervous system.

Surges of adrenalin and cortisol energize and prepare our body for action. We breathe faster and our heart rate increases. In a highly threatened state, we may feel more inhibiting responses in our body, such as freeze (feeling paralyzed), or appease (becoming submissive). These are our "tricky" brain's way of protecting us.

Drive-excitement system

The drive system stimulates positive feelings motivating us to acquire resources and achieve goals. For example, feelings of pleasure linked to falling in love, consuming food, and achieving at work. These all release the hormone dopamine, boosting our sense of achievement and self-esteem.

What can jeopardize the drive system is when it interacts with threat. Those driven to work hard due to a fear of failure, or who constantly engage in "doing" mode to avoid being with their feelings, throw their emotional system out of balance. Mothers are often in "doing" mode, juggling caring for their baby with domestic tasks and the

Drive system
Stimulates positive
feelings.

Soothing system
Helps us feel
content and connected.

Threat-
focused system
Prepares our body to
fight, flee, freeze,
or appease.

maternal mental load (*see p186*). Overactivating this system leads to exhaustion and burn out.

Soothing system

When we're not defending against threats or busy achieving, our soothing system switches on, helping us feel calm. Feeling safe dials down our threat system. Our brains have evolved to respond to nurturing, yet this system is often neglected in people—including tired new moms. Accessing our "rest and digest" system facilitates attachment and a sense of inner peace.

Just as regulating our baby through rocking, stroking, and gentle words strengthens their soothing system, consider it a muscle that needs flexing for us, too. Compassion is about giving and receiving kindness, and an important part of this is learning to soothe ourselves. Our soothing system allows us to "mentalize"—to tend to our own emotions, as well as imagine what our baby might be feeling.

Affirmations and Visualizations

Practicing mindful compassion teaches you a kinder, stronger relationship with yourself. Compassionate visualizations and affirmations activate your soothing system—grounding you, and, in turn, your baby.

A Buddhist view of compassion draws on the metaphor of the lotus flower in the mud. The mud is your suffering—difficult, painful feelings and thoughts, which understandably you want to run away from. But the lotus flower needs the mud to grow. So to really understand suffering means descending into the mud and acknowledging and tending to painful parts of you, without judgment.

Self-soothing

Regular mindful compassion strengthens your "thinking" brain's abilities, allowing you to bring awareness to intense tidal waves of emotion. You learn to recognize signs that waves are building, finding ways to connect to safety instead of being swept away by the tides. You can then choose wisely how to respond.

"Let go of the struggle against anxiety, anger, and sadness, to free you to bloom as a mother."

The visualization exercises here will help you cultivate your compassionate self through mindful awareness of strong feelings without judgment (*see p80*), quieting your inner critic (*see p126*). Practice self-soothing with affirmations and imagery to calm your anxious or angry self, as you recognize and make room for difficult emotions (*see p170* and *p172*). These exercises switch on your soothing system—allowing you to be fully present with your baby and to tend to their strong feelings as they arise. They also teach you self-forgiveness and self-acceptance in becoming the mother you want to be (*see p188*).

The benefits

Mindfully focusing on what you're grateful for has many benefits, including stronger relationships and feeling happier, healthier, and more hopeful. Crucially for moms—gratitude helps you cope with stress (*see p114*).

Research shows that half hour daily practice over just eight weeks leads to brain changes in people who have never practiced compassion. Doing regular loving-kindness meditations can change your genes (*see p76*). This is an ongoing journey as parenthood inevitably shifts you into threat mode—yet with practice, you can change your brain and genetics.

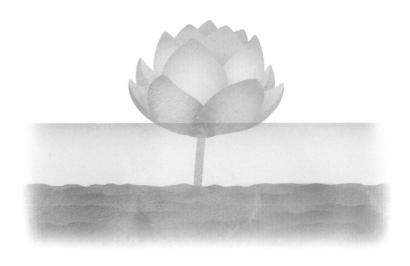

Breathing and Meditation

The stresses of motherhood can cause moms to ricochet between "threat" and "doing" mode. Use your breath as an anchor to bring calm, clarity, and a renewed energy to caring for your baby.

It's easy to feel overloaded amid all the relentless, daily tasks, when you're bone tired and unsure whether you're getting it "right." Moments of overwhelm, whether linked to your baby crying or worry about the never-ending to-do list, trigger a strong physiological reaction in your body (*see p20*). In threat mode, you breathe shallowly. You shift out of your ability to "be" with your experience. You may become consumed with negative thoughts such as "I'm not good enough"

or "My baby's so difficult." Perhaps you berate yourself for feeling low, anxious, or angry because of messages internalized about how "good" mothers should feel. This creates shame— fueling the negative cycle of thoughts, feelings, and bodily sensations.

So how do you break this cycle? As psychiatrist and psychotherapist Viktor Frankl says, "Between stimulus and response, there is a space. In that space is our power to choose our response. In our response lies our growth and our

"*Use your breath to calm, restoring your ability to think, so you can respond mindfully to your baby.*"

SOOTHING RHYTHM BREATHING

This is slower and deeper than normal breathing, stimulating your soothing system and moving you into "being" mode.

Lengthen your spine, soften your face, and gently focus on your breath. Breathe in with purpose, counting to three on the inhale. Pause, then count to three on the exhale. The idea is to elongate each inhale and exhale, finding a rhythm and pace that suits you. Once you've found a sense of stillness, lengthen the exhale. Count to three on each inhale, then to six on each exhale. Elongating the exhale activates your relaxation response, soothing difficult thoughts and feelings.

freedom." A simple yet powerful way to create that space is to focus mindfully on the breath. This isn't to say you can breathe all your problems away. But as the breath connects your conscious and unconscious—uniting your mind, body, and emotions—you can use it to regulate your nervous system.

Breathing

Directing your attention to your breath, for example, when your baby is crying, allows you to pause. Conscious breathing calms mental spirals of overwhelm, creating mental space and restoring your ability to think. The short, practical exercises in this book will help you self-regulate in moments

of stress. You can also use soothing rhythm breathing (above) as your go-to practice, to help you settle into a meditation, affirmation, or visualization as you go about your day. Try this breathing technique when you make your coffee, take your baby outside (*see p116*), or before feeding (*see p90*).

Meditation

You may wonder why this book suggests meditation for new moms when you already have so much to do. Stress zaps precious emotional energy, and in a culture that glorifies busyness, it's vital to give your brain and body a chance to relax—to relieve stress and reset your nervous system. Conversely,

»

inducing a relaxed state (even if only for 5 to 10 minutes) reenergizes you. This is about reframing self-care. Bookending the day with short meditations isn't selfish or lazy; it's crucial for your sense of self, allowing you to replenish your capacity cup before it spills over. Claiming this time for yourself takes active effort—no one else will do it for you. Following these exercises actively switches on your soothing system, offering you headspace and containment, in turn benefiting your baby.

The idea that meditation means clearing the mind is a myth. Our brain and body are always in flow—thoughts, emotions, and bodily sensations fluctuate in intensity. Whether sitting for a brief meditation (*see p54*) or enjoying everyday mindful moments (*see p72* and *p82*), you become more awake and attuned to your inner world. Mindfully directing attention inward allows you to attend to whatever arises, without judgment. This includes noticing any painful feelings and sensations. While unpleasant, you will come to view thoughts as "mental events"—acknowledging these with kindness and letting them go. Your "tricky" brain is simply trying to protect you. You also learn that painful emotions and bodily sensations are ever-changing—like waves, they peak in intensity yet always come down. You learn to trust your ability to ride out these feelings. They won't destroy you. Meditation teaches you to understand and nurture your emotions instead of fighting or cutting off from them. Instead of reacting, you can choose to respond compassionately, both for yourself and your baby.

Benefits of meditation

Cumulative benefits of meditation include strengthening areas of the brain linked to emotional regulation and empathy, such as the prefrontal cortex, hippocampus, and insula (*see p12*). These positive brain changes have been found to significantly benefit emotional and physical health, increasing flexibility of attention and acceptance. Research shows that meditation supports sleep quality, boosts mood and well-being, and reduces rates of depression. One study found that meditation reduced negative mood, which related to learning to be curious about difficult feelings.

Note of caution

If you find focusing attention on your breath or body distressing, due to difficult bodily experiences or triggering strong feelings, start by focusing attention outward to the space around you (*see p116*). If you continue to experience regular moments of overwhelm, speak to someone you trust and reach out for support (*see p214*).

"Meditation will bring a spaciousness and confidence to your mothering role."

27

Natural Remedies

These natural remedies and rituals, many of which draw on ancient wisdom, will help you feel nurtured, nourished, and looked after. Therapeutic and holistic, these remedies place maternal well-being at their center.

We are not designed to raise our baby in isolation, yet mothers in Western cultures often do. The safe, natural remedies in this book would have, in years gone by, been passed down by grandmothers living close by. Some remedies can be used alongside medical options; others you may find more deeply therapeutic because they offer greater holistic care. Be sure to discuss options with your healthcare practitioner first.

Learning to prioritize yourself is essential for your recovery and sense of self as a mother, as well as being of benefit to your baby. Cultivate a compassionate, mindful approach to yourself to help your body heal and to sustain you emotionally amid the stresses and strains of parenting.

Optimal perineal care

After the birth, make your own pain-relieving padsicles to soothe vaginal bruising and soreness (*see p94*). A couple of days postpartum, entrust your baby to the care of your partner or a dependable friend while you relax in a warm, herbal bath to promote perineal healing (*see p99*).

"These remedies are about personal choice—select the best for you."

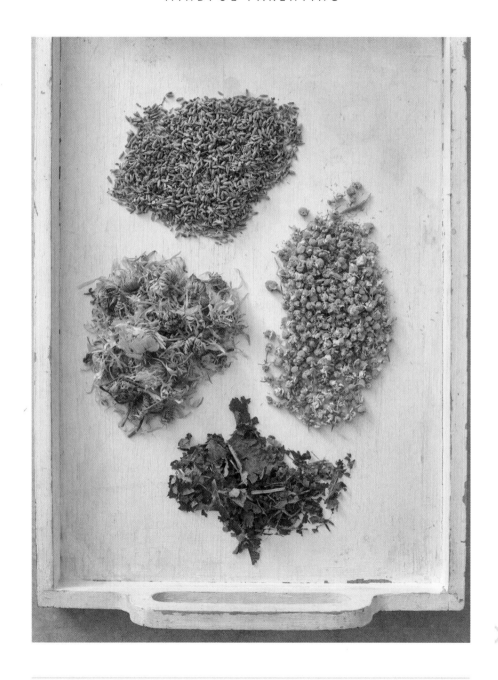

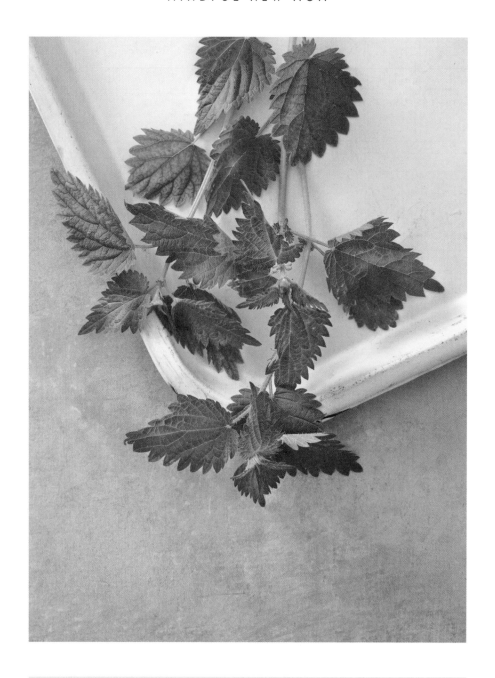

"Honor your need to replenish reserves and prioritize yourself."

Postpartum care

Many new moms feel apprehensive about their first bowel movement postbirth, and psyllium powder is a natural stool softener (*see p56*). To manage any anxiety, tune in to your soothing rhythm breathing (*see p25*), as this will relax your pelvic floor.

Cold packs, cool witch hazel, and herbal baths can all help reduce inflammation and shrink hemorrhoids (*see p94* and *p99*). Consider liquid tonics to boost energy levels following blood loss. These are a good alternative to solid supplements (*see p56*).

Breastfeeding remedies

You will experience noticeable changes to your breasts as your milk comes in, including engorgement, where your breasts feel very hard and full. Cool Savoy cabbage leaves placed on your breasts can ease discomfort (*see p56*), along with frequent feeding to relieve engorgement.

Aromatherapy oils

To cope when you are feeling overwhelmed, use essential oils to ground yourself (*see p132*). You can draw on your mindfulness skills and use your breath as an anchor (*see p25*), while inhaling the scent of your chosen essential oil on a handkerchief. As your baby grows, you will find small pockets of "me" time begin to open up. If you have a partner, put aside some time to reconnect through touch, using a unique blend of aromatherapy oils for a sensory massage (*see p196*).

Promoting sleep

Disrupted sleep is part and parcel of motherhood, but that doesn't mean simply accepting exhaustion as your lot. Prioritize rest when you can and create nurturing rituals before bed to help you relax (*see p165*). This may include drinking a calming herbal tea (*see p118*) or using soothing essential oils (*see p165*).

Movement- and Nature-based Practices

Movement is medicine, shifting us out of our heads and into our bodies. Mindfully connecting to nature, particularly immersion in water, helps us heal and detoxify, reducing stress and enhancing mood.

Adjusting to the emotional ups and downs of parenting can be tough. Alongside the joy and wonder, stressors such as sleep deprivation, isolation, feeding challenges, and "ghosts in the nursery" (*see p151*) can trigger difficult feelings. Since suppressing these feelings uses up valuable emotional energy, we need to consciously connect to how our feelings are felt in our bodies.

When we become aware that emotions are linked to physical sensations, we can listen to our bodies. Bodily awareness frees you to pause and make wise choices to respond to your needs—whether resting, mindful eating, walking, swimming, or saying "no" to something you don't prioritize. This tuning in takes practice, and you may feel disconnected from your body after giving birth.

"Experiencing weightlessness in water feels so freeing in contrast to the physicality of mothering."

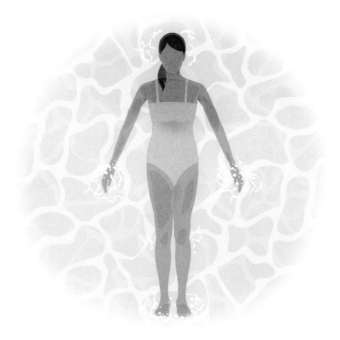

Mindfulness teaches us to attend to our internal experience, acknowledging the wisdom of our body; it tells so much of our suffering. We learn to nurture strong feelings with compassion and kindness.

Blue therapy

Immersion in water can bring calm, boost focus and well-being, lower anxiety, stimulate creativity, improve sleep quality, and reduce pain. Even just looking at pictures of the sea, or visualizing it in your mind as your "Special Place" (*see p134*), is soothing.

Swimming is a great low-impact exercise. If you can tolerate low temperatures, chilly dipping plunges you right into the present moment. Even just splashing your face with icy water can activate your soothing system (*see p168*). Cold water swimming is believed to have many benefits, including reducing anxiety, boosting mood and immunity, and focusing attention on the breath, body, and surrounding space. A sense of achievement and euphoric high usually follow as you emerge, body shivering, buzzing, and tingling.

Green therapy

Getting outdoors is the surest way to lift energy and mood—for you and your baby. Abundant evidence highlights the emotional and physical benefits of accessing green spaces—so take a meditative walk in nature (*see p116*).

Being in natural settings helps us destress—and quickly. Only four to six minutes of contact with natural versus urban spaces significantly restores relaxation. Sensory awareness is heightened and attention and focus enhanced. Green exercise therapy, including gardening and walking, has many mental health benefits, such as boosting confidence and self-esteem. Even viewing greenery in a photo acts as a soothing, healing balm.

Yoga

You may feel your body isn't quite your own at this point, but gentle yoga postures will help you regain trust in your body, supporting a kinder

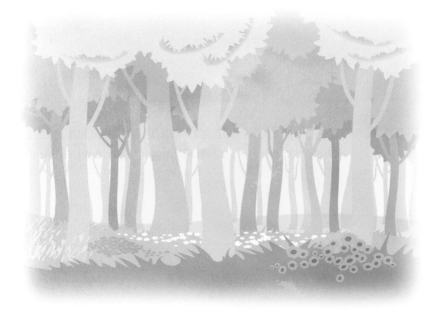

"Connecting to nature will help you destress—soothing your nervous system."

relationship with it. Every sequence in this book has been adapted for each postpartum stage; tailor the sequences according to what fits for you. You could begin by doing several poses of the first sequence (*see pp138–145*) and, as you regain energy, add in a couple more. These poses are designed to support flexibility, core strength, and focus. Postures such as the Lying Down Twist (*see p177*) will help counter tension in your back and shoulders.

Protecting even just 10 minutes of peace on your yoga mat is a powerful way to bring calm and come into your body. Mindful breathing creates space to listen to what's going on internally, soothing your nervous system, allowing you to reset. Using your breath as an anchor will help you disidentify from unwanted thoughts (*see p25*).

The restorative poses encourage you to nourish your soothing system. Inverted poses such as Legs Up the Wall (*see p181*) are beneficial for your heart and rebalancing your energy. The Side-lying Pose (*see p145*) is a lovely way to rest while feeding your baby.

Baby massage

Respectful touch through baby massage creates an embodied connection. Sensitive stroking turns on the soothing system in you both, producing oxytocin and feelings of calm and connection. In Asia, baby massage is a well-established mothering ritual, and it has become more popular in Western cultures.

Parents widely report positive benefits of baby massage, including feeling more relaxed, closer to their baby, and more confident in reading cues. Studies have also shown benefits of massaging preterm babies in neonatal wards. It's also a lovely way for partners or grandparents to bond with your little one (*see pp102–107*).

Nutrition

The process of creating and birthing a baby places huge demands on your body, depleting you of nutrients and reserves. Choose nutrient-rich, energy-giving, and mood-boosting foods to help you regain your strength.

This life-changing transition can take a toll on your body—depriving it of key micronutrients (vitamins and minerals), and macronutrients (proteins, carbohydrates, and fats). Add in hormonal shifts, stress, and sleep deprivation, and you have a recipe for postpartum depletion.

Mindful approach to food

The first three months, known as the "fourth trimester," is a time to cocoon with your newborn—not only for their benefit but also for yours. Resist Western expectations to "bounce back" postbirth effortlessly and unsupported. Our ancestors would have raised children in groups. New mothers learned from their elders, drawing on their wisdom and support, an approach that continues today in collectivist cultures. These cultures allow time for the mother to rest and heal, away from day-to-day pressures (*see p78*). New moms are also nourished with a special diet of nutrient-dense foods.

"A mindful approach to eating means listening to your body and making wise, nutritious choices."

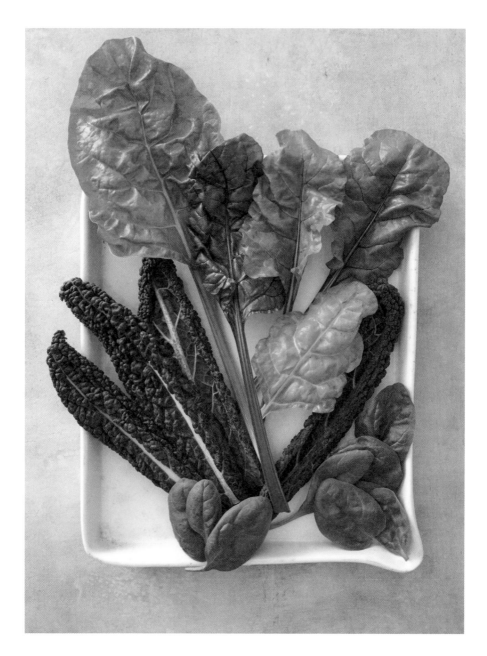

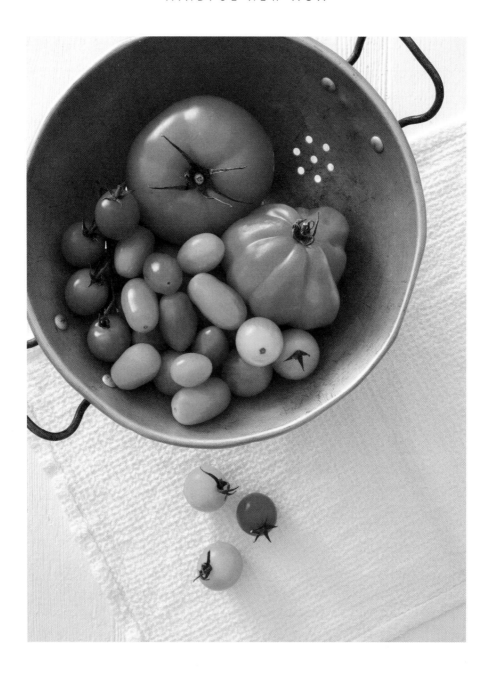

"Draw on Eastern traditions that honor postpartum care and respect and nourish new mothers."

Nourish body and brain

In the days following birth, draw on Asian traditions by warming your body with nourishing soups and protein-rich bone broth to aid healing (*see p52*).

Enjoy the "rainbow" of fruit and vegetables, such as kiwifruit, red berries, peppers, and spinach, to help replace lost nutrients (*see p52*). You also need to replenish levels of iron following blood loss during birth (*see p74*). Remember to drink plenty of water to stay well hydrated.

Balanced diet

For a healthy, balanced postpartum diet, you need good sources of calcium and protein (*see p88*); slow-release carbs; healthy fats; and fiber (*see p52*), to sustain energy levels.

Breastfeeding is beneficial for your baby, but it can deplete you of important nutrients. Rebuild key vitamins into your diet, including vitamins A, C, and E (*see p85*).

Eating well

Stress and lack of sleep play havoc with your mood and energy levels. Avoid skipping meals—your blood sugar levels will dip, leaving you feeling depleted, as if your cup is about to overspill. Eating mindfully means listening to your body when you're hungry or thirsty and prioritizing your needs (*see p122*). Make a sandwich or have healthy snacks on hand to eat before tending to your baby—even if they're crying. You'll need the energy to comfort them!

Choosing foods rich in tryptophan, such as turkey, and magnesium, such as avocados and legumes, can enhance your mood and well-being (*see p129*). For optimum long-term health, shop and cook mindfully (*see p191*).

Connecting to Values

Your values act as a compass, guiding you on your mothering journey. They empower you to face challenges and make decisions, helping you feel rewarded and fulfilled in your role as a parent.

What kind of mother do you hope to be? This may be a tricky question to answer, as you're just embarking on your parenting odyssey. But it's a useful question to reflect on as part of this life-changing transition, whether this is your first, second, third, or last baby. Your core values connect to what gives you meaning and purpose in life—to what you really care about.

Research shows that living a life in line with your values nourishes your emotional well-being. Return to the idea of yourself as an oak tree: imagine your values are your branches, intrinsic to who you are and what matters to you. Some of these branches are big, while others may be less visible. All these branches represent what you hold most precious in life—your hopes, beliefs, and actions that help you flourish and feed your preferred stories of identity.

Using the values exercises

The reflective exercises in this book support you to explore your mothering

"Ask yourself: what small action can I initiate today to become the mother I want to be?"

values (*see p136*) and illuminate branches that may have temporarily slipped out of view. Connecting to your values empowers you to use your maternal intuition for making all the complex decisions that mothers face each day. It allows you to feel more at peace with your mothering style, helping you discern what advice to discard and what to accept (*see p130*).

Selecting your core values

Pick out five or six values that you hold dear (see below for ideas). The values you pick are your guiding branches— these help you feel centered and at one with yourself. Values aren't goals but ongoing actions that give life purpose. In challenging times, you may need to be flexible with them. Try staying true to your values in a good-enough way.

CORE VALUES

Connection	Power	Friendships
Contribution	Tradition	Love
Trust	Adventure	Growth
Creativity	Spirituality	Justice
Family	Community	Kindness
Equality	Authenticity	Respect
Recognition	Fun	Wisdom

WELCOMING YOUR BABY

Birth is a momentous event, and the first 48 hours after welcoming your baby bring a constellation of intense emotions. Grounding affirmations will anchor you as you adjust to your new role as a mother and help you enjoy mutual soothing with your baby. You'll also find invaluable advice to nourish your postbirth body.

The First Few Days

After meeting your new baby, you may feel a whirlwind of intense emotions. You may feel elated, relieved, happy, proud, and overcome with love. You may also feel numb, exhausted, disappointed, and tearful.

Mothers are expected to feel a rush of natural love toward their newborn based on the myth that bonding comes naturally. In reality, we know nearly half of first-time moms report feelings of indifference—sometimes due to sheer exhaustion. Remember, it takes time to get to know your baby.

Whether you've had a vaginal or Cesarean delivery, birth is a monumental event. Immediately afterward, you may experience physical sensations such as shaking or nausea as adrenalin leaves the body, particularly after a difficult birth. It's normal to feel preoccupied with yourself after such a visceral experience.

A mindful approach postbirth means acknowledging all the feelings as they arise, using your breath to anchor you during waves of panic or overwhelm. Use grounding statements and personal objects (*see p50*) to manage any emotional surges

"*You may feel raw and vulnerable after the birth. As your baby is born, so too are you as a mother.*"

following the delivery. Along with affirmations for acknowledging difficult feelings if your birth didn't go as planned (*see p62*), these mindful techniques will encourage gentleness with yourself as you adapt to your new role.

The first hour

The first hour after birth offers an intimate and important (but not essential) time for bonding. Your body is still home to your baby, as you welcome them in your arms right away. Most newborns placed on the mother have the amazing ability to "breast crawl" to the nipple to begin feeding. This suckling floods both you and your baby with oxytocin, allowing you to gaze at each other, infusing you with mutual feelings of love and wonder. Later, when your milk comes in, the hormone prolactin signals the release of milk, bringing feelings of calm and contentment.

Initial bonding with your baby

From the moment your baby arrives, they are wired for connection. You both begin the "dance of interaction": your baby is primed to feel calmed or engaged by cues such as your facial expression, eye contact, and the

66 99 A MOTHER'S STORY

I was absolutely terrified when we came home. Those first few days all feel like a blur now. I remember feeling so elated but also so raw, emotional, and exposed. In between the shock, pain, and joy, I was really concerned with making sure Nina was safe. I was worried about doing anything wrong. I was obsessed with making sure she was swaddled properly and the temperature in our room was just right. It really started to consume me. The sleep deprivation, sore nipples, pain from my episiotomy, pinched nerves—it really was so much to manage, even though I had good support from the midwives and my family. Yet despite the fear, there were also moments of absolute wonder and joy.

Amber, mother of Nina

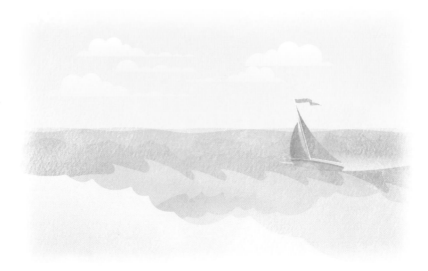

familiar sound of your voice. The breathing meditation on page 54 can help you find synchronicity with your baby during this special time.

Skin-to-skin bonding

Creating a mindful pause for skin-to-skin bonding will benefit you by enhancing closeness with your baby. Skin-to-skin contact also facilitates breastfeeding and reduces rates of depression. This proximity benefits your baby, too, by regulating their breathing, body temperature, and nervous system. If you are unable to have skin-to-skin contact, don't worry. There are plenty of opportunities to

bond with your baby through touch and being mindfully connected (*see p54*). It's never too late.

Emotional changes

In the early days, as you become totally focused on your new baby, you may feel highly emotional and protective. This state of heightened awareness, known as "primary maternal preoccupation," allows you to tune in to your baby and respond sensitively to their needs. However, feeling so at one with your baby can be overwhelming at times, filling you with anxiety and urgency when, for example, they cry. It can even create tension between you and your partner if your partner feels excluded. It can be reassuring to know that this intense preoccupation, which can feel all-consuming, is temporary and entirely normal.

Physical changes

As well as the emotional and hormonal upheaval, birth also has a huge impact on your body. Physiologically, you may be experiencing pain and discomfort, especially if you've had an episiotomy, tearing, or stitches. After a Cesarean section, which is major abdominal surgery, anything involving your stomach muscles such as sitting, rolling over, and walking, can hurt. Along with appropriate pain relief, arnica tablets are commonly taken to promote healing and reduce any swelling (*see p56*).

No matter how you gave birth, heavy vaginal bleeding is common in the first few days as your body sheds the lining of the uterus. Stock up on maternity pads and make sure your diet is rich in iron (*see p74*) as your iron levels will be depleted by blood loss.

You may also experience afterpains as your uterine muscles contract back to their prepregnancy size following the birth. Try mindful breathing (*see p60*) to help manage the pain.

Time to recuperate

It takes time for the body to heal after birth, particularly if it was traumatic. If you feel you missed out on the birth you hoped for, or weren't shown kindness and respect and need further help or advice, see page 214.

In Western cultures, the expectation is for adjustment after birth to be quick and seamless. Elsewhere, postpartum practices recognize the need for maternal recuperation, so bring a kind acceptance to yourself at this time.

"Lower expectations at this intimate and unique time and don't be afraid to ask for help."

Meeting Your Baby

After the primal physicality of birth, the moment you have waited for has finally come. Savor the intimacy of those first few minutes meeting your precious new baby. Appreciate the wonder of this new life you have created.

1

Bring a heartful open presence to this little person that you will come to know. With feelings of awe, relief, and tenderness, rest your gaze softly on your baby's face. Bring a soft smile of gratitude to this peaceful moment.

2

Notice your baby's fine features. Look lovingly into their beautiful eyes slowly opening up to their new world. Feel the smooth satin of their skin.

3

Wonder at their delicate fingers and tiny toes. Breathe in the sweet scent as they rest in your arms.

4

Tune in to any sounds they are making. Speak softly to them, soothing them with your gentle words. They are familiar with your voice from being in the womb. Sing a song they may know from their life living inside you.

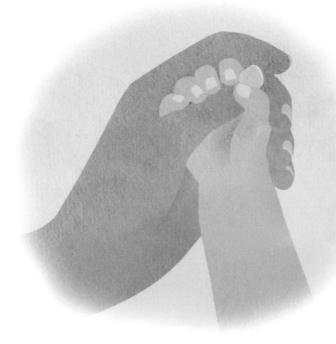

5

Marvel at the miracle that is your baby. Feel the aliveness of this moment-to-moment connection flowing between you. Allow yourself to absorb the quiet intensity of your shared stillness. Pause and appreciate that you have created this tiny baby.

6

Be open to what your baby will teach you on this parenting odyssey you will travel on together. And trust that you will tap in to your own inner wisdom as you go. Drink in the beauty of this moment and make a mindful intention to take each day as it comes.

Managing Intense Emotions

Whether your baby is born in the hospital or at home, ensure you have your sensory self-soothing tool kit close at hand. Affirmations and grounding objects can help you cope with the adrenalin-fueled moments postbirth.

1

Mindfully create a cocoon of calm for you and your baby.

2

If at home, keep the lights low or use candles. Ask your birth partner to regularly plump up your pillows and listen to your birth playlist or ambient music.

3

If in the hospital, take LED candles to create a soothing glow and headphones to listen to peaceful music. Don't forget comfy pillows plus an eye mask and earplugs. You could also take a photo of loved ones.

4

Keep your favorite perfume or essential oil, perhaps jasmine or lavender, or a scented handkerchief near you. Breathe in the familiar scent to ground you in moments when you may feel overwhelmed.

5

Draw on affirmations to ground you if a surge of panic or overwhelm arises. Name your feelings. Try visualizing them as waves—rather than resisting the waves, you can learn to surf them.

6

Gently say self-soothing statements to yourself. These will help calm you, relaxing both body and mind. Choose your own statements or use the ones below.

"When these waves come, they're unpleasant— but they will pass."

"I'm feeling _____ (name the emotion[s]), and I am safe."

"It is normal to feel intense feelings at this time. It's going to be okay."

Nourishing Postpartum Foods

At a time when you are focusing on your baby, cultivating compassion for yourself is vital for your recovery. Making mindful choices about the food you eat plays a key role in rebuilding your strength.

Making sure you are eating fresh, nutrient-dense foods will help you recover physically as well as give you the energy you need to care for your baby. Don't forget to drink plenty of **water** and stay well hydrated, especially if you're breastfeeding. To boost physical healing, collagen-rich **bone broth** fortifies your body with amino acids. This protein-packed broth is especially beneficial for tissue repair, helping your body cope with sleep deprivation and stress after childbirth.

To ease postpartum constipation—a common complaint among new mothers—make sure you eat plenty of fiber. Aim for 30 grams a day by "eating the rainbow" of fruits and vegetables, for example, **kiwifruit**, **apples**, **strawberries**, **raspberries**, and **cantaloupe** (*see right*). You can add **peppers**, **carrots**, or **spinach** to stews or salads or sprinkle ground **flaxseed** on oatmeal.

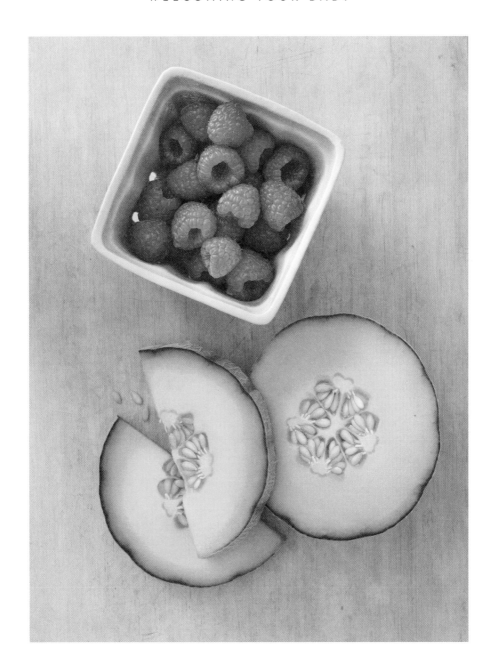

The Mother-Baby Bubble

Create a bubble with your new baby for skin-to-skin cuddles. Follow this meditation when your baby is quiet to calm both your heart rates, bringing mindful awareness to mutual soothing.

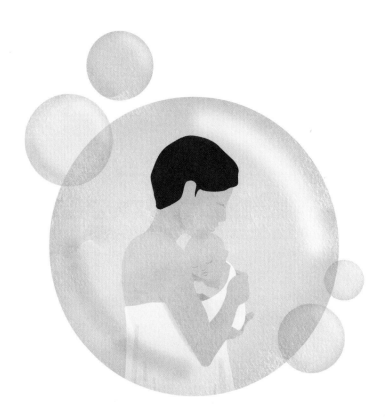

1

Make yourself comfortable with your baby, skin-to-skin. Take deep, relaxing breaths and soften your face.

2

Drop your shoulders as you allow your mind and body to settle. Bring your attention to your breathing. Notice where you most easily feel or sense the breath.

3

Feel the warm weight of your baby lying on you, skin-to-skin. Notice how their little body lifts with each inhale. And then with each exhale, notice their body fall in synchrony with yours.

4

Try to match your rhythm of breath to theirs. To support a sense of gentle presence, mentally say the word "calm" on the inhale. Then, with each exhale, say the word "ease."

5

Thoughts and feelings may come and go. Your mind may feel jumpy and scattered. That's okay. Gently guide your attention back to your breath. Continue to enjoy this closeness with your baby as it brings them comfort.

6

Take these warm, relaxed feelings with you for the rest of the day. Repeat at any time to soothe you both.

Healing Postpartum Remedies

Your body has undergone an extraordinary event. Common postpartum discomforts include perineal soreness, constipation, and breast engorgement. Try these soothing remedies to promote healing.

The process of labor and birth can place strain on your digestive system, leading to constipation or trapped wind. Sprinkle a teaspoon of **psyllium powder** into a glass of water as a natural stool softener. To restore energy levels following blood loss during birth, **liquid tonics**—containing organic iron, herbs, and vitamins—are preferable to solid supplements. To ease perineal discomfort, **arnica tablets** are a popular herbal remedy for reducing inflammation.

After a couple of days, the volume of milk coming in can make your breasts feel swollen, hard, and hot. Frequent feeding relieves engorgement, along with applying cold cabbage leaf compresses to the breasts. Wash and refrigerate green **Savoy cabbage** leaves (*see right*). When needed, place the leaves over the engorged area for up to 20 minutes. Don't leave them on for longer as they can dry up milk supply.

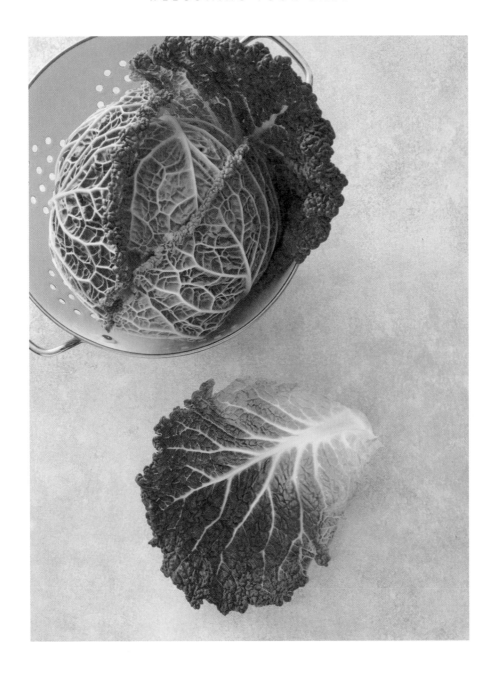

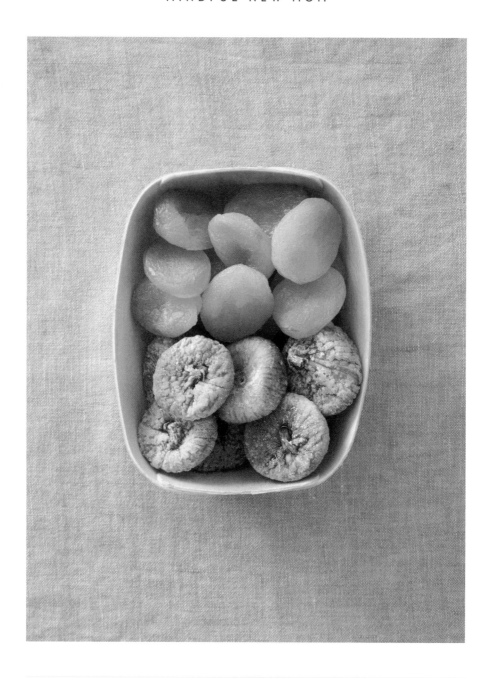

Sustaining Postbirth Foods

During labor, eating may well have been the last thing on your mind, so you may find yourself ravenous after giving birth. Honor your accomplishment by treating yourself to your favorite foods.

Many women say that the first food they eat after giving birth tastes the best they've ever had. Your celebratory postbirth meal doesn't need to be fancy, but it's an opportunity to reward yourself. Ideally, pack delicious and nutritious snacks in your hospital bag. Naturally sweet **dates** or **dried figs** or **apricots** (*see left*) are good options. Keep portions relatively modest, as eating little and often, drinking plenty of fluids, and snacking on fibrous foods helps aid digestion.

You may have missed certain foods during pregnancy, such as raw fish, rare meat, or runny eggs. If it can be organized, you will relish every mouthful of that long-awaited **sushi** or rare-cooked **steak**! Try to make one of your first meals at home a special one. Choose foods that will replenish your body with good-quality protein and nutrients such as iron (*see p74*).

Exploring Birth Pains

Mindfully exploring your relationship with pain helps you respond differently to intense physical sensations. Follow this breathing meditation to cope with afterpains or for surgery-related discomfort.

1

Think about the three components of pain: the sensory component (bodily pain sensations), the emotional component (how you feel in relation to the pain), and the cognitive component (mental talk or images).

2

Bring your attention to your breath. Notice whether your attention is pulled to any challenging sensations and see if you can name them. Any tightening, aching, or throbbing? Notice where the sensations are most acute.

3

Bring a kind and open curiosity to these sensations. You may notice they are not fixed but continually changing.

4

If waves of discomfort continue, say to yourself gently: "I welcome these sensations as a sign of what I've achieved in birthing my baby. These life-giving pains will pass, eventually."

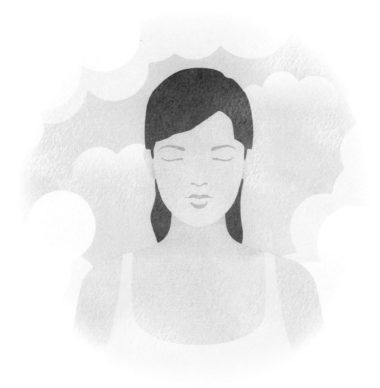

5

You may experience negative mental talk or images, or feelings of resistance to the pain. Just notice whatever comes up, without judgment.

6

Guide your attention back to your breath. Count "one" on the inhale and "two" on the exhale. As you exhale, feel a sense of releasing and letting go.

Making Sense of the Unexpected

Not having the birth you hoped for, or experiencing a difficult birth, can leave you feeling vulnerable right at the start of your parenting journey. What matters most is acknowledging and tending to your feelings.

1

If choices were taken away from you, you may be left feeling disappointed, guilty, or like a failure. Whether you felt unsupported, frightened, or lacking a voice, remember this was never your fault.

2

Honor and make space for any intense emotions as they arise. If you feel tearful, allow yourself to cry. If you feel numb, acknowledge these feelings with kindness.

3

Imagine that you, along with every new mother, have been gifted a knapsack. This bag is heavy, weighed down with difficult feelings such as guilt and shame. Guilt can be driven by impossible expectations falling so heavily on women—no wonder your knapsack is hard to lift!

4

On your journey, you'll need to unpack your knapsack. Try talking to others. Understanding guilty feelings can help lighten your load.

5

When you can't find the words, try these soothing affirmations to remind yourself how well you're doing and how far you've come.

"My baby and I did the best we could. It wasn't easy, but I coped, and we are together."

"It wasn't my fault my birth didn't go as planned. I am not a failure."

"I have brought my baby into the world. I am amazing. I am enough."

"I will heal, in time."

"I am just what my baby needs."

COCOONING WITH YOUR BABY

Allow yourself to cocoon with your baby in the first six weeks. During this special time, use natural remedies, nutritional advice, and yoga to heal and fortify your body. Establishing feeding can bring challenges, so use meditation to help you cope. If you're struggling, reach out for support.

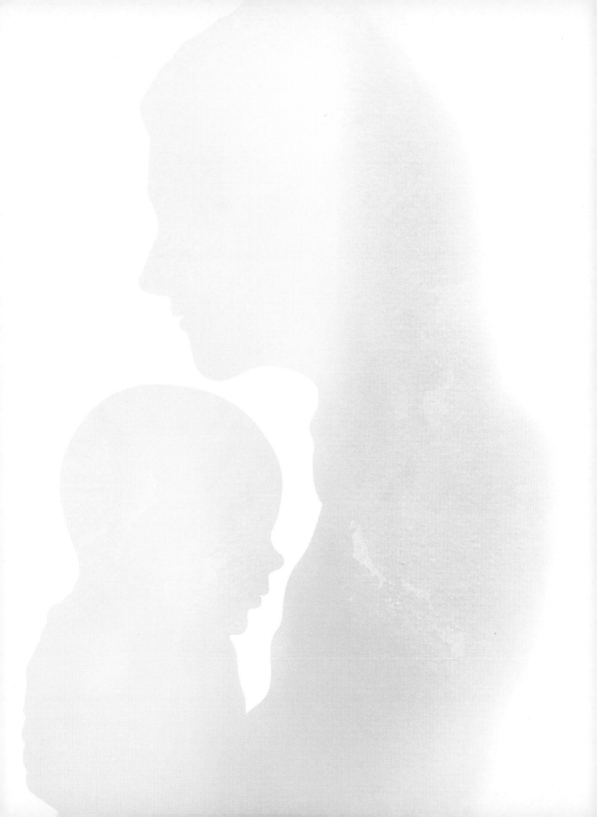

Cocooning with Your Baby

The early weeks can feel like an emotional roller coaster as you adjust to life with your newborn. It's important to remember that it takes time for your body to heal, and this period is about giving yourself permission to rest.

Try to let go of any pressure to be up and doing things. You're still recovering from the physical aftermath of birth, while learning the ropes for all the "doing" of mothering. Consider the fourth trimester as an opportunity to recuperate and cocoon with your baby, either in bed or your feeding zen zone (*see p86*), to recreate womblike warmth and closeness.

It may feel like life has been turned upside down, as if you've entered some other-worldly place. Some days you may manage to actually leave the house with your baby; other days you may not even shower and get dressed. Go gently. It's normal to feel up and down, especially given hormone fluctuations and broken sleep.

The first weeks

The early days can be exhausting. And yet, aside from all the practical mothering tasks, you may secretly wonder what it is you're doing all day at home with your baby. This chapter introduces important ideas related to containment and the "dance of reciprocity" that should reassure you that you're doing *far* from nothing.

From the moment your baby is born, they communicate with you in every way they can. You may feel like a novice detective, desperately trying to decipher any clues in that cry, gurgle, frown, stretch, and, soon, smile. Are they hungry? Needing comfort? Too cold? In pain? Babies come into the world full of powerful, tumultuous feelings and physical states. They need your help to make sense of their confusing, contradictory inner feelings as they adjust to their new outer world.

Feeding

Establishing feeding during the early weeks takes up energy, both physically and emotionally. If you're struggling to breastfeed, remember to try skin-to-skin with your baby. Studies show that this close contact increases success rates. Some initial discomfort during feeds is common (*see p101*); this may relate to anxiety, which can create tension. Try natural remedies (*see p56*) and meditation (*see p90*) to help.

You may feel heartbroken if, for all sorts of valid reasons, you're not able to breastfeed. However, there are many other opportunities to bond with your baby, for example, through baby massage (*see p102*), where you tune in and sensitively respond to your baby's cues. This is a key part of reciprocity as you and your baby interact and actively try to be in step with each other.

Struggling to breastfeed can often feel like a failure on the mother's part, but it really is about both mom and baby learning the way together. Learning to recognize your baby's cues takes time. Adopt an Observer position, be curious, and follow your baby's lead.

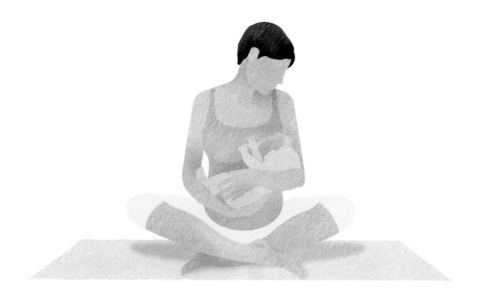

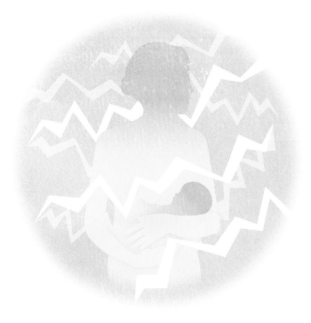

Containment

Containment is when you "hold" and then process your baby's intense emotions—without becoming overwhelmed yourself. You then "give back" your baby's intolerable feelings in a more digestible form. This process allows your baby to feel heard and understood, soothed and safe. For example, when your baby cries, you might say: "Poor you, I can hear you're upset. Mommy's here, and it's okay."

Physically holding your baby helps them feel contained, too. Sometimes babies cry frantically when they are undressed because they feel so vulnerable, as if they're "falling to pieces." You may have already found that wrapping them up close in your arms helps them feel safe and secure. Through holding, rocking, a gentle voice tone, and reassuring facial expressions, you calm their big, scary feelings. All these loving actions turn on your baby's soothing system. Providing a safe haven for your baby is an important part of attachment, allowing them to develop a sense of self, and, over time, the ability to soothe themselves.

Of course, all this containing impacts your emotional capacity. As with the oxygen mask analogy (*see p18*), in order for you to feel with your baby, you need to be able to soothe yourself or your head will just become too full. We all have different limits for when our capacity cup spills over, depending on our own unique stressors and experiences. It can be especially hard as a single parent, or if you're managing a health condition, a child with disabilities, or multiple children. If you feel moments of overwhelm are so frequent that they're preventing you from enjoying everyday life with your baby, talk to someone you trust. Containing your baby means learning to separate out which feelings "belong" to you as the mother and which "belong" to your baby. This takes a lot of emotional energy, especially when sleep deprived!

Being supported

So who holds you as the mother? Given levels of parental isolation, mindfully creating your own Circle of Support is vital to help you feel contained (*see p78*). Giving yourself permission to rest and take time for yourself is also important for your sanity and self-esteem. This could be offloading to

66 99 A MOTHER'S STORY

Feeding was the hardest thing I faced as a new mom. I was determined to breastfeed because I'd read about the benefits, but I knew it wasn't always easy. For the first couple of weeks, my nipples were so sore and there was barely any milk. My son was impatient when he was hungry and would scream if the milk didn't come out fast enough, so I often bottle fed. My parents used to get frustrated with me for persisting with breastfeeding and a few times I called a helpline crying. When my second child came, it was totally different. He latched on right away, and there was plenty of milk.

Sital, mother of Kishan and Rishi

"Getting help early shows strength and a commitment to improving things for you and your baby."

a loved one, doing a short meditation (*see p76*), taking time to have a relaxing herbal bath (*see p98*), or reminding yourself of soothing affirmations (*see p96*). These are all ways to calm your nervous system and help your head feel less full.

Triggers for vulnerability

Motherhood can tap into and trigger vulnerable parts of us that may have been unconsciously packed away—especially when coping with major brain and body changes, plus hormonal fluctuations. We all come to motherhood with our own ideas and stories. Our individual contexts, such as cultural expectations, childhood experiences, trauma, adversity, difficulties conceiving, baby loss, and experiences of feeling "othered" (for example, related to race, class, and sexuality), can all increase vulnerability.

Speaking up

The notion of "Supermom" creates the idea that as moms we *ought* to know—so it can be really hard to reach out for help. Many women worry that sharing their feelings honestly will lead to being judged a bad or unfit mom—or worse, having their baby taken away. These fears can present real barriers to new mothers speaking out.

Trusting in others

Practicing mindful compassion offers a helpful, forgiving way to anchor yourself in the tumultuous early period. But it's also important to call on trusted friends, family, and health professionals who can help you make sense of your experiences. Quality of support is key, so make sure those you ask are supportive and not critical or undermining. For advice on seeking help, see opposite and page 214.

RECOGNIZING EMOTIONAL DIFFICULTIES

Motherhood can push you to your limits, but struggling doesn't make you a bad mother. It is crucial to understand why you may be feeling this way and seek support so you can get help.

Birth trauma

One in three women experience some aspect of birth as traumatic, upsetting, and/or frightening. You may experience flashbacks, nightmares, or intrusive memories of the birth and avoid any reminders of it.

Baby blues

Most women experience the "baby blues" around three to four days after giving birth, due to hormonal changes. You may feel tearful, low in mood, and anxious. Difficulties beyond the first two weeks should be taken seriously.

Postpartum psychosis (PP)

This is a severe but rare condition affecting around one in 1,000 women. Signs include mania, hallucinations, anxiety, and delusions. PP is considered a medical emergency but is treatable if recognized.

Postpartum depression (PPD)

More than one in 10 women experience PPD in the first year after birth. Signs include low mood, thoughts of hurting yourself, feeling overwhelmed, numb, and worthless. Risk factors include feeling unsupported, a history of depression, high stress, and a difficult birth.

Postpartum anxiety (PPA)

More than one in 10 women experience PPA, which can occur alongside PPD. Signs include persistent feelings of tension or fearing the worst. Perinatal Obsessive Compulsive Disorder (OCD) involves experiencing recurring thoughts or obsessions.

Postpartum rage

A symptom of PPD, the signs of postpartum rage include struggling to control temper, violent thoughts or urges, and negative feelings or little interest in baby. Anger can mask grief and fear, yet "good" moms may suppress it due to shame. Risk factors include lack of support, inequality, and trauma.

Mindful Dance of Attunement

Offering a mindful presence to your baby when they're relaxed brings great opportunities for connection. Shift out of "doing" mode and into "being" mode by slowing the tempo and being open to what your baby brings.

1

Choose a time when your baby is well fed, warm, dry, and comfortable. Ensure you, too, feel relaxed. Offer an inviting presence, with your shoulders relaxed and chest open, so your baby feels safe.

2

Give your baby a soft smile and observe them. Wonder what they might be feeling.

3

Speak warmly to your baby. Name what you think they may be thinking or feeling. Over time, naming their emotions helps them understand their feelings.

4

If your baby communicates by gurgling, facial movements, or a gesture, show them that you've noticed. Respond with loving words, smiles, and a warm gaze.

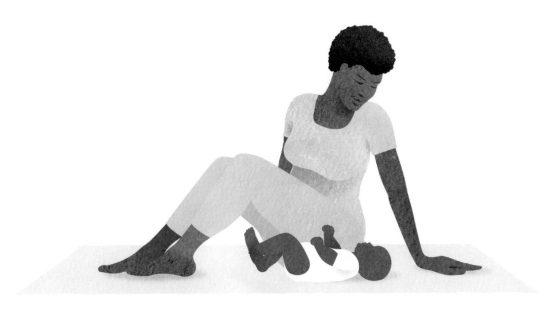

5

Again, watch your baby. This is turn-taking in action as you step back, observe, and tune in to your baby's signals, and then respond in kind— maybe mirroring their actions.

6

If your baby turns their head away or yawns, this is simply a sign they need a break after moments of connection. All this interaction is tiring—they'll come back to you when they are ready.

7

Wait, watch, and observe once more. Initially, these interactions could last a few minutes. As your baby grows, notice obvious and subtle changes in this mindful dance of attunement.

Energy-boosting Foods

Tiredness and low energy are very common in the early days. Blood loss leaves many new mothers low in iron, which can result in fatigue. A varied mindful diet will help boost energy levels.

Iron is required for healthy red blood cell production. If you are deficient in iron, your body will not get enough oxygen, resulting in low energy. For a delicious iron-rich meal, eat **steak** or **lamb** with wilted **spinach**. Although less easily absorbed, plant-based sources of iron, including **fortified cereals**, **dark leafy greens**, **beans**, **lentils**, **nuts**, and **tofu**, are great, nutrient-rich alternatives. To increase absorption, pair your iron sources with a good source of vitamin C such as a glass of **orange juice**.

Try to eat balanced meals to sustain energy levels. Combine slow-release carbohydrates such as **sweet potatoes** and **whole grain pasta** with lean protein such as **chicken** or **cod**. Include healthy fats such as **avocados** (*see right*), **eggs**, **nuts**, and **oily fish** as well as good sources of fiber such as **broccoli**, **tomatoes**, or **hummus**.

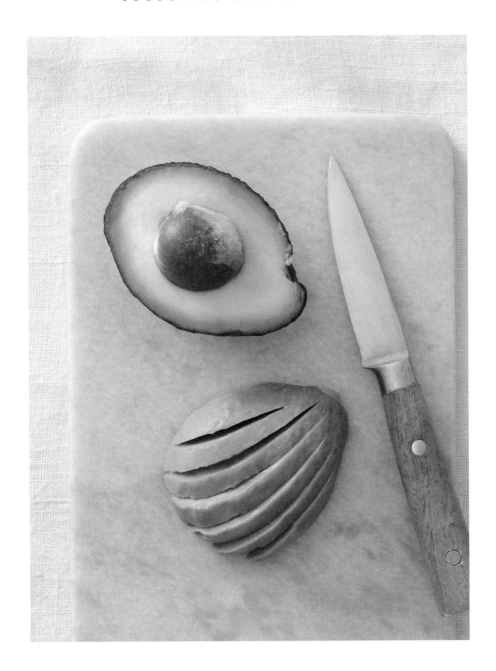

Loving-kindness Meditation

As you adjust to parenthood, your threat system will be on high alert. Acknowledge your desire to protect your precious baby. Practice loving-kindness as an antidote to intense fears that come with your love.

1

Focus on your breath. Rest a hand on your heart, inviting feelings of warmth.

2

Direct the following phrases softly to your baby:

May you be safe and healthy.
May you be loved.
May you be joyful.
May you be at peace.

3

Notice any thoughts, emotions, or sensations that arise. You may feel a deep sense of love and gratitude for your new baby. Bring awareness to any difficult feelings, too, without judgment.

4

Now focus on you, saying:

May I be safe and healthy.
May I be loved.
May I be joyful.
May I be at peace.

5

Appreciate that
you, too, need the
same love and care as
your baby. Try holding
a picture of you
as a baby, repeating
the phrases.

6

Send loving-kindness
outward to people
in your life who have
supported you.
Direct the phrases
to loved ones
and mentors.

7

Finally, extend
the circle of loving-
kindness to all human
beings. Recognizing
our common
humanity, repeat
those phrases again.

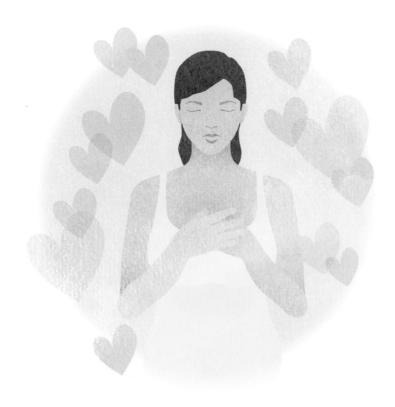

Reflecting on Your Circle of Support

An African proverb states, "It takes a village to raise a child." Yet in Western cultures, parents are often less connected to their wider networks. Mindfully creating your own circle of support will allow you to recuperate.

Tasks such as feeding, changing, and bathing, along with soothing your baby day and night, can make your head feel very "full." You are still recovering physically, and adjusting to the new demands and responsibilities of motherhood can feel overwhelming—this is completely normal. In order to contain your baby, it's important to think about who is containing *you*—whether it's your partner (if you have one), extended family, or wider support system.

Initially, you may feel very focused on your baby, and it can feel hard to ask for help and take care of yourself. You may also feel anxious about handing your baby over to someone else. Sometimes people feel undeserving of help or see it as a sign of failure. If this applies to you, the first step is bringing mindful awareness to this struggle. Try reframing an offer of help as an opportunity to get the optimum care for you and your family.

CREATING A CIRCLE OF SUPPORT

Draw or visualize an innermost circle for you and your baby (and maybe your partner), surrounded by an inner circle and then an outer circle. Figure out who fits where within the circles.

You and your baby

Place you and your baby in the innermost circle, as this time is very much centered around you both. You will hopefully be enjoying regular rest as you recover.

You and your closest support

You may wish to place your partner or closest support in the innermost circle with you, depending on how supported you feel. Their role is to protect your mother-and-baby bubble.

Emotional closeness

Reflect on those you trust, who don't judge you—these are the people you can be vulnerable with. These trusted members of your tribe truly listen, allowing you to offload and process your feelings. Consider where to place them, in the inner or outer circle.

Social support

Social support is key to you feeling contained during this vulnerable time. Consider who you share a sense of ease with. Social support can be offered by a trusted health professional, too. Position people offering social support in the outer circle.

Practical help

For practical support, borrow from non-Western postpartum practices by enlisting helpers to relieve you of hands-on tasks. The emphasis is on helpers, rather than visitors who take up energy. Place these helpers in the outer circle.

Connecting to Your Compassionate Self

Consider the three flows of compassion: kindness from you to others; kindness you receive from others; and kindness you show yourself. Focus on creating your own wise, soothing, inner "compassionate self."

1

Showing yourself compassion may feel alien. If so, imagine you've been cast as an actor in a movie—try becoming the character of your compassionate self.

2

To embody the confident, steady presence of a compassionate person, visualize yourself as an ancient oak tree, rooted firmly in the ground, exuding confidence and ease.

3

Sit down and direct your attention to your breath. Breathe into your belly with purpose. Focus on lengthening each inhale and each exhale.

4

Soften your face. Bring a gentle friendliness to your facial expression. Imagine speaking to someone kindly, saying, "I am here for you."

5

Reflect on the qualities of compassion. Imagine your compassionate self feeling a sense of responsibility—moving away from blame and judgment. This mentor wishes only to guide you through challenges, to help you move forward and grow.

6

Connect to your compassionate self when you feel you've got it wrong. Reframe regret—as you learning to be a mom.

7

Consider soothing actions your compassionate self will take. Perhaps running a bath for you or giving you permission to nap. This strong, wise part of you recognizes what you need, bringing encouragement and understanding. Remember, even if you don't feel these qualities, the most important thing is your mindful intention to strengthen your soothing system.

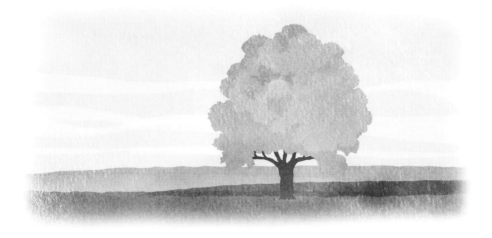

One-minute Mindfulness

You may find yourself performing the hands-on tasks of mothering on autopilot. Redirecting your attention in this 60-second practice wakes you up to the present, as a human "being," not a human "doing."

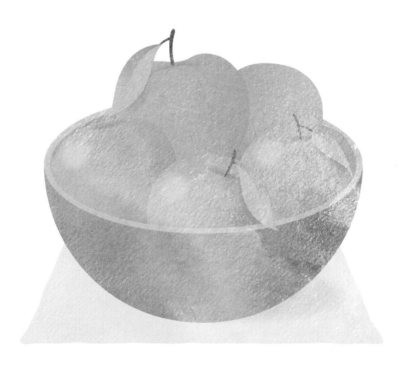

"We often rush eating or eat mindlessly; instead, take time to really savor your food."

1

Explore an apple in the way your baby might, with fascination, awe, and wonder.

2

Notice the colors of the skin you can **see**—look for any different shades or bruised areas.

3

Feel its weight in your hand. Notice the texture, whether it feels smooth and shiny or uneven.

4

Put the apple next to your nostrils and breathe in its **smell**. Just be curious about the aroma.

5

As you bite with intention into the apple, tune in to the different **sounds** this action creates.

6

Bring awareness to the **taste** as you chew slowly. Notice any sensations in your mouth after you swallow.

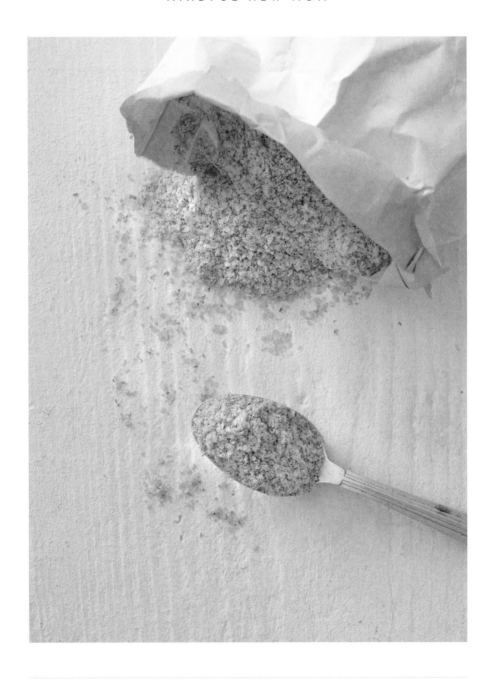

Replenishing Postpartum Foods

Pregnancy, birth, and breastfeeding all require high levels of micronutrients to feed your body. To avoid postpartum depletion, choose natural foods so that you replace key nutrients and support your immune system.

Make sure you have a vitamin-rich diet. Vitamin E is an important fat-soluble vitamin and antioxidant found in **eggs**, **leafy green vegetables**, **nuts**, and **sunflower seeds**. For an easy vitamin E boost, sprinkle **wheat germ** (*see left*) over oatmeal or include in a smoothie. Vitamin A strengthens immune function and is found in foods such as **spinach**, **carrots**, and **sweet potatoes**. Eat plenty of **citrus fruit** and **berries** to maximize your intake of vitamin C, a key antioxidant that supports the immune system and aids your body's healing process. Also consider taking a vitamin D supplement as the primary source of this vitamin is sunshine, and deficiencies are common.

"Make nutritious choices to nurture and enhance long-term health."

A Zen Feeding Zone

Mindfully make a zen zone for feeding, with all your creature comforts on hand to nurture you as you nourish your baby. Take refuge in this quiet space for a chance to pause, breathe, and reconnect.

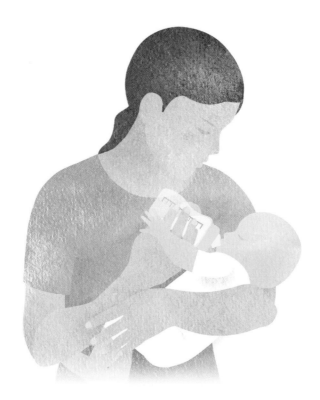

1

Creating an oasis of calm at home will encourage you to relax, in turn soothing your baby. Be mindful that you're shifting from "doing" to "being" mode, building peaceful associations for both of you.

2

Whether you are breast-, bottle, or mixed feeding, ensure your "nest" has everything you need. Which key elements will reinforce a sense of calm? Perhaps a comfy feeding chair or a cozy blanket to keep you both warm.

3

Within arm's reach, have muslins, a magazine or book, and your phone. Keep water and healthy snacks nearby.

4

Before each feed, take a moment to ground yourself. Even if your baby is becoming agitated, use your breath and body to anchor you to *this* moment. Take a couple of deep breaths into your belly. Feel the soles of your feet on the floor. Notice how supported you feel in your chair.

5

Feel your baby's warm body in your arms as they anticipate being fed. Drink in their delicious smell. Meet their loving gaze and notice any sounds of satisfaction. Allow your breath to find its natural rhythm, enjoying these moments of mutual connection—flooding you both with oxytocin.

Optimum Foods When Breastfeeding

If you're breastfeeding, your baby will get everything they need from your breast milk. Ensuring that you eat a diet high in protein and calcium and that you are well hydrated can promote milk production.

Protein is key for your baby's growth and development, as well as keeping your muscles, bones, teeth, and tissues healthy. Aim for three good-quality sources of protein a day. Animal sources of protein such as **meat**, **fish**, **dairy products**, and **eggs** contain all the essential amino acids; or for good vegetarian or vegan sources, eat **soy products** or a variety of plant-based sources such as **beans**, **lentils**, **nuts**, and **seeds**.

Calcium is essential not only for building your baby's bones but also for maintaining your bone density. Aim for four to five rich sources of calcium every day. Calcium is found in **milk**, **cheese** (*see right*), and other **dairy products**. Plant-based sources include **fortified milk**, **cheese alternatives**, **bread**, **cereals**, and **dried fruit**. To increase calcium levels, enjoy a **yogurt** for breakfast, snack on **almonds**, and combine **sardines** with steamed **broccoli** for a healthy lunch.

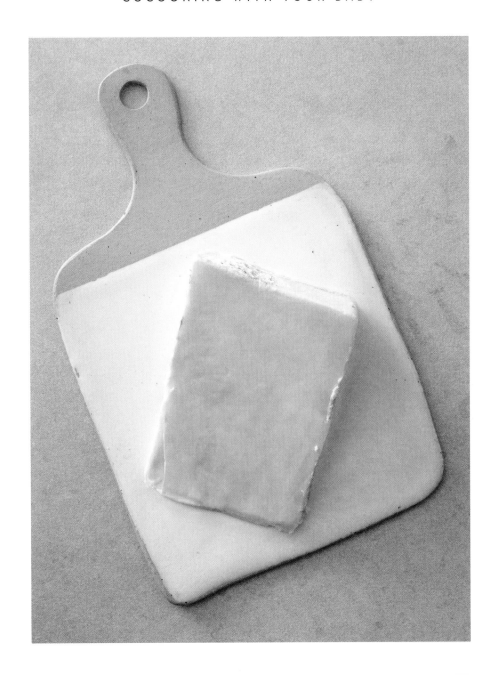

Mindful Feeding

The idea that breastfeeding comes naturally is a myth. In reality, it takes time, and discomfort is common initially as you and your baby learn together. Being mindful can help alleviate tension that can intensify pain.

1

Feed in a quiet space such as in bed or your zen zone (*see p86*) to build calm associations for you and your baby.

2

Take a few deep breaths. Draw your shoulders back and sit so you are well supported. Soften your jaw.

3

Imagine a flower opening between your eyebrows. It's not easy, but the more relaxed you can be, the more your baby will be, too.

4

As your baby starts sucking, notice any sensations in your body. Note how you respond to any twinges, perhaps related to the let-down reflex, or soreness.

5

You may find yourself reacting to strong sensations by tensing your body or face. You may also berate yourself with harsh self-judgments such as "I'm failing."

6

It's natural to react strongly to pain and wish it away. Yet this aversion can increase suffering. See if you can label all sensations as "passing events." Notice their ever-changing nature.

7

Whenever the sensations become too distracting, direct your attention back to the breath. Mentally say the word "Calm" on every inhale. On each exhale, say the word "Ease." Notice any tension melting away.

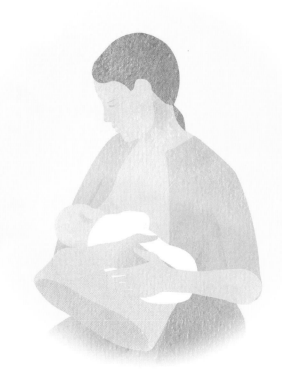

Pelvic Floor Awareness

Regain the strength of your pelvic floor with these awareness exercises, coupled with mindful breathing. If you're in physical discomfort, begin by practicing them as a visualization, then progress to the movements.

1

Sit up tall with a straight back. Take a deep breath in. As you breathe out, draw up your back passage internally, then follow that engagement forward and up. Imagine a line from your tailbone to your navel, and softly draw those two points toward each other.

2

Engaging your pelvic floor is an internal lift—it doesn't involve any other muscles. Relax your bottom, thighs, shoulders, and jaw.

3

Try not to hold your breath. Focus on timing the squeeze-and-lift with an exhale, then allow the entire pelvic floor to relax on the inhale. Practice several times, exhaling slowly as if blowing out a candle.

4

Repeat with intention three times a day. Practice while doing tasks such as picking up your baby, lifting a car seat, or lowering your baby into the bath, as all these activities use your core.

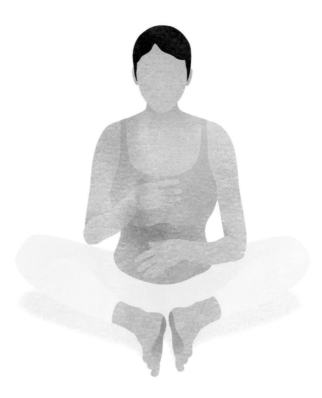

5
—
Each time you
lift your baby,
consciously breathe
out and draw up into
your pelvic floor.

6
—
Practice releasing your pelvic floor with
deep, slow abdominal breaths into the lower
belly. This will stimulate your soothing
system and release tension, bringing a sense
of calm to the chaos of early motherhood.

Padsicles for Perineal Healing

Soothe vaginal bruising, swelling, and soreness with postpartum padsicles. Combining the effects of a pad and an ice pack, these frozen maternity pads are full of natural healing properties to help ease pain.

To prepare your maternity pads, presoak with **alcohol-free witch hazel** to reduce inflammation. Rub pure aloe vera gel over the pad using clean fingers. **Aloe vera** (*see right*) has anti-inflammatory and analgesic properties. You can also apply a few drops of essential oils such as **lavender** or **rosemary** to your pad to calm swelling and fight infection. Store in the freezer for at least an hour before use, allowing to thaw a little before wrapping in a washcloth to avoid the pad coming into direct contact with your skin. Apply the padsicle for up to 30 minutes at a time for immediate relief.

"Padsicles will feel especially soothing in the first few days after birth."

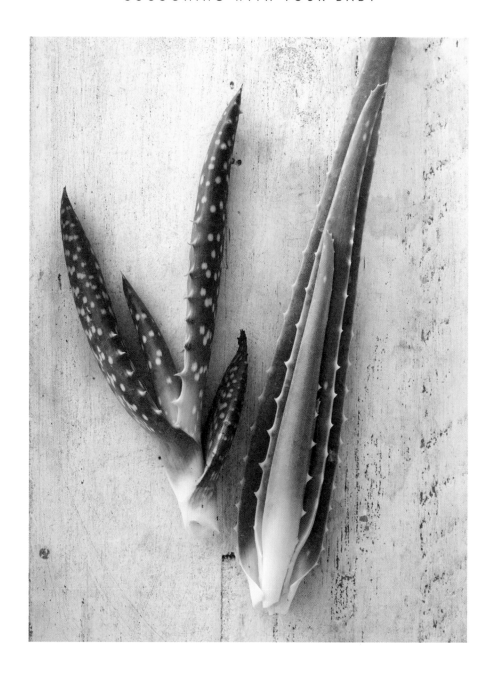

"SPACE" Affirmation

The challenges of feeding while coping with broken sleep and your own physical recovery can trigger moments of overwhelm. Bring compassionate awareness to these moments through this soothing practice.

1

Soothing rhythm breathing

Focus on deepening your breath, inhaling for three counts and then exhaling smoothly for three counts. On each exhale, notice a sense of slowing down.

2

Posture

Embody the dignified, open presence of your compassionate self. Sit with your back straight, dropping your shoulders and opening your chest. Relax your face and neck.

3

Acknowledging

Place your hand on your heart, asking yourself tenderly: "How am I feeling right now?" Acknowledge any feelings of anxiety, anger, or sadness with kindness.

4

Compassion

Compassion means making space for all the different parts of you. Tune in to and acknowledge any fears, sensations, and critical thoughts.

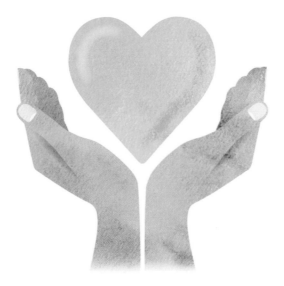

5

Empathy

Learning to shine a compassionate light on your thoughts and feelings in stressful moments allows you to take an Observer position. Imagine yourself as a caring pilot hovering over these difficult inner experiences. This creates space for you to step back and respond wisely and kindly.

6

Name your feelings, telling yourself gently:

"I'm having a stress reaction. I'm feeling _____ (insert emotions) and I'm safe."

Next, allow your compassionate self to soothe you. Practice saying these statements out loud in a gentle voice:

"These feelings will pass."

"I'm a good enough mom. I *can* cope."

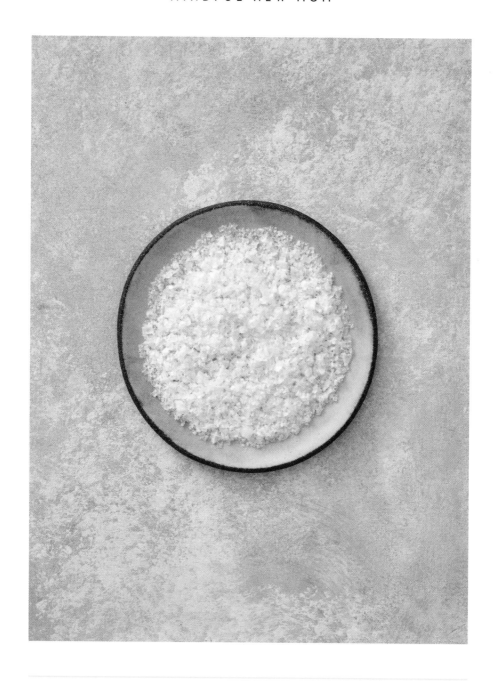

Healing Herbal Bath

A soothing, healing herbal bath is a wonderful opportunity to relax undisturbed while helping your body recover from soreness and swelling. If you aren't ready for a full bath, a sitz batch can relieve discomfort.

Choose herbs that are soothing and healing as well as antibacterial and anti-inflammatory. For each muslin bag, combine 9oz (250g) of **unrefined sea salt** (*see left*) and 2oz (50g) each of **lavender flowers**, **witch hazel flowers**, **calendula flowers**, and **chamomile flowers** (all of which can be bought online). Drop one bag into a hot bath, infusing your bathroom with gorgeous scents. Once the bath has cooled to a comfortable temperature, immerse yourself for a relaxing, healing soak.

Adding essential oils to a warm bath provides relief as well as healing. Speak to a health professional first, as some wounds may need to stay dry for longer. Mix 3–12 drops of **lavender oil**, which is antiseptic and calming, and **tea tree oil**, which helps fight infection, in a tablespoon of carrier oil. Stir the bath before stepping in. Alternatively, add some flakes of soothing **magnesium**.

Accepting Professional Support

Finding a trusted professional source of help is important if you feel you are struggling with breastfeeding or emotionally or with your physical recovery postbirth.

Every new mother should receive a six-week OB or midwife check for her physical and mental health, and this is an important chance to answer any doubts you have or ask for help. As appointments often feel rushed, it is worth thinking about what you want to discuss beforehand. Prepare to advocate for support if you need it. Six weeks allows the first stage of soft tissue healing. Remember, even if you're "signed off" at your check, it can take longer for your abdominal and pelvic muscles to recover. Just because you're deemed "safe" to resume exercise and sexual activity, it may be a while before you feel ready.

"Hold onto hope. You will find your sense of self again."

ACCEPTING PROFESSIONAL SUPPORT

If you are finding aspects of motherhood difficult, don't delay in reaching out for help as things can spiral quickly. For advice on where to get help, see page 214.

Breastfeeding

Concerns about your baby's latch when breastfeeding, or persistent pain beyond the first week or so, can indicate support is needed. This could be from a registered lactation consultant, breastfeeding counselor, or a national helpline.

Physical recovery

At your six-week check, mention anything that doesn't seem quite right. Pain and lack of sensation are not "normal." Incontinence or flatulence can indicate pelvic floor dysfunction; feeling heaviness in your vagina can indicate prolapse; abdominal separation (diastasis recti) can affect pelvic floor function.

Emotional well-being

Be open and discuss the degree of distress you are experiencing. Note how long your emotional difficulties have been going on for, intensity (how much they get in the way of your sense of self and everyday life), and frequency.

Help for physical issues

If you have concerns, ask to be referred to a women's health physiotherapist who can do a full musculoskeletal and internal examination.

Help for emotional issues

Speak to an empathetic family member or friend and consider what you might say to a health professional. The OB's role is to get you the best help and refer you if necessary.

Practice and Techniques

Sensitive touch is key to our emotional survival—even baby monkeys need tactile comfort to feel safe. Infant massage is a gentle way to get more in touch with your baby, helping you both feel calmer and more connected.

Babies respond to sensitive touch from birth, but you may want to start more formal practice after the very early weeks when they could find it too stimulating. Choose a time when they're content and alert, not too soon after feeding and when your baby isn't tired or hungry. Stroke rhythmically, applying moderate pressure, and be mindful of cues that they've had enough, such as crying or retracting their legs or feet. Do not use any oils until after the first month (or longer in premature babies), when the top layer of skin has sufficiently developed. Olive oil is not recommended, but you could use other cold-pressed oils, ideally organic and unscented.

"Talk or sing softly to your baby as you massage them, letting them know they are loved."

10-MINUTE MASSAGE SEQUENCE

*An important part of infant massage is stroking your baby
with sensitivity and respect. At first, start with just one or
two of the massages, then, as they get used to being massaged,
build up to the full sequence and increase the duration.*

01

THUMB OVER THUMB

Ask permission before undressing your baby. Lie them on a towel in a warm room and remove their clothes (and diaper, if you wish). Sit so you can make eye contact. Hold your baby's foot and, using your thumbs, gently stroke your baby's foot from heel to toe. Watch as your baby's toes uncurl. Wait for their toes to straighten, then repeat the massage stroke. Repeat on each foot as many times as your baby seems to enjoy.

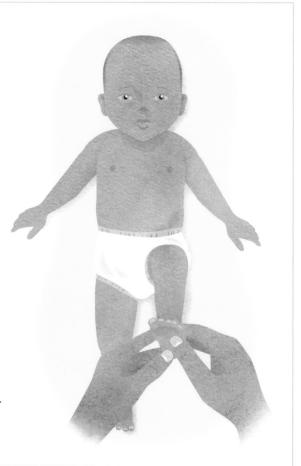

»

02

MILKING

Wrap your hands around your baby's thigh and gently draw down from the thigh to calf, hand over hand, as if "milking" the leg. Repeat as many times as your baby seems to enjoy, then switch and repeat on the other leg. Talk to your baby as you massage their legs.

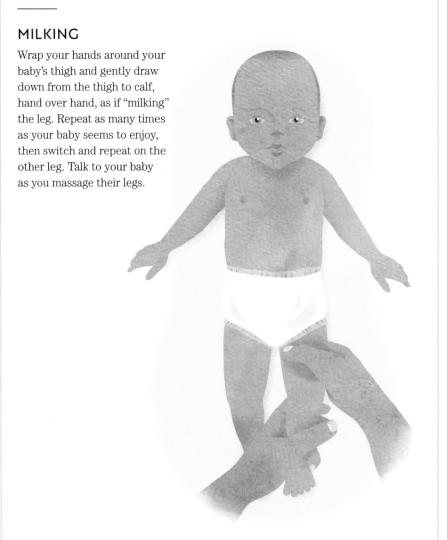

03

SAUSAGE ROLL

Raise your baby's leg and roll their thigh gently between your palms, moving down to the calf, then carefully return their leg to the floor. Repeat as many times as your baby seems to enjoy, then switch and repeat on the other leg.

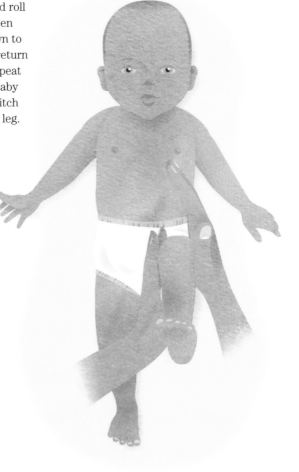

>>

04

FACIAL MASSAGE

This massage is good for easing teething-related pain. Focus on your baby's face, making sure you are careful of sensitive areas. Actively trace little circles on their cheeks. Then trace little circles below their lower lip and repeat above the upper lip. Pull their earlobes gently as these have pressure points connecting to the mouth.

05

FLATTENING THE PAGES OF A BOOK

Place two fingers (the index and middle fingers of each hand) on your baby's chest on each side of their sternum and gently stroke outward. Lift your fingers, return to the start position, and repeat as many times as your baby seems to enjoy.

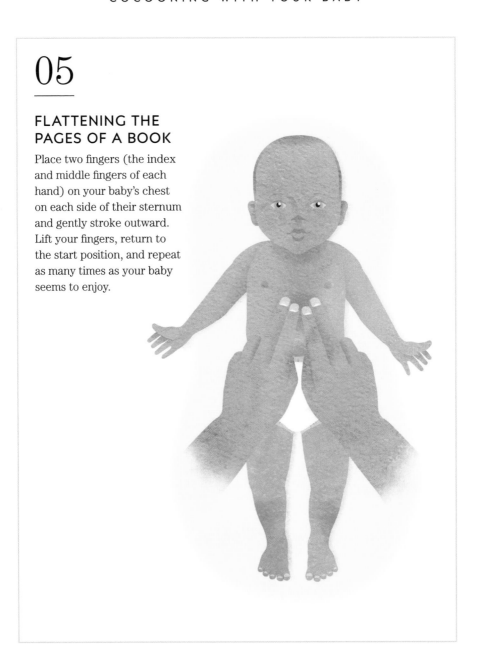

ADJUSTING TO LIFE WITH YOUR BABY

*Weeks six to 12 can feel exhausting—
try to surrender to this intimate time,
enjoying those newborn snuggles.
Amid "Supermom" expectations and
your inner critic, use meditations,
affirmations, and imagery to recenter
you, along with mindful walking and
gentle yoga. Identify your values
to tap into your inner wisdom.*

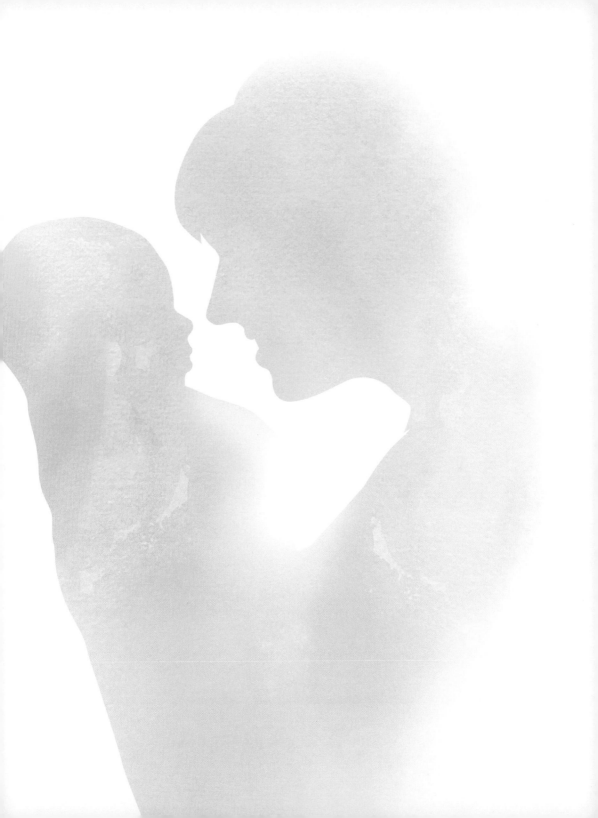

Adjusting to Life with Your Baby

Being a mindful mom can help you create mental space amid the mayhem of the first months, allowing you to tune in to your intuition, connect with your values, and truly own your parenting choices.

As your newborn develops, use mindfulness to savor special moments of snuggles. Take time out amid the often chaotic day to appreciate the wonder of this new little person in the world. Try practicing gratitude to help you celebrate "small wins" (*see p114*) and mindfully connect to music as you sing your baby to sleep (*see p126*).

From the moment your baby arrives, you are bombarded with advice. This begins in pregnancy, when so much is dictated to you. Then, after the birth, you're the one in charge. Yet it can feel like all the expert voices, whether from medicine, the media, or well-meaning relatives, are so loud.

All the conflicting, often unsolicited, advice about mothering is confusing.

What unites these often opposing agendas is that they prescribe a "right" way to parent. This creates anxiety for many mothers, especially given that your baby hasn't read the manuals. As psychotherapist Naomi Stadlen points out, it can feel like you've entered a war zone, where you feel defensive no matter what choices you make.

Adopting a mindful approach
Recent research shows how common negative thoughts are in new mothers: nearly two in three nondepressed moms reported thinking, "I am a bad mother." Yet the more negative thoughts they had, the more they felt guilt and shame—because these thoughts don't seem to fit the "good"

mother ideal. Recognizing and observing your inner critic—the harsh internal voice that berates you for your actions and mothering choices—is a key step in mindfulness (*see p126*). Find ways to ground yourself, such as connecting to nature (*see p116*) or soothing with essential oils (*see p132*).

Practicing ways to recenter yourself is especially important in these early weeks, when your baby requires so much of you. The peak age for crying is around six to eight weeks. Babies often become fractious and overstimulated after all the sensory input of the day. Breastfed babies also tend to cluster feed, which is exhausting. Try to

surrender to it—get comfortable on the sofa and enlist others to give you a break. During the day, protect small pockets of time to soothe stress and relieve tension by practicing a few calming yoga poses (*see p138*).

The myth of "Supermom"

What lies at the heart of parenting pressure is society's focus on perfection. Sometimes referred to as the perfect mother myth, the Supermom myth, promoting the fantasy mom as martyr, runs deep. Supermom shapes our expectations of motherhood—placing huge pressure on moms to live up to an impossible ideal. It leads to

»

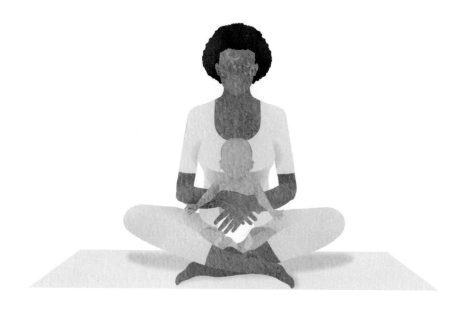

moms believing they must prove to themselves and the world that they are calm, coping, and cherishing every moment, even if they aren't. In reality, Supermom sets mothers up to fail.

Caring for your baby brings many magical, tender moments, but the messy, tiring, repetitive nature of the fourth trimester can come as a shock. We know that babies can stir all kinds of feelings in us, linked to our own unique past experiences. Yet Supermom doesn't allow any negative feelings, silencing women. In aspiring to be a "good" mom, women put on a brave face, hiding their anxiety, anger, or sadness. Efforts to uphold these "masks of motherhood" only make moms feel as if everyone else is coping, leaving them feeling even more alone.

Diminishing Supermom

Bringing mindful awareness to the impossible Supermom expectations allows you to release yourself—so you can make wise choices from a more forgiving place. Stepping back allows you to notice negative judgments from others. Usually, however, the biggest source of judgment is yourself.

66 99 A MOTHER'S STORY

Despite being a very friendly and active person, I felt a certain sense of isolation and loneliness in not conforming. I learned that there is a standard way of doing things, and that not following certain unspoken rules could make even the most confident parent feel insecure. Not conforming to the norms made me feel embarrassed, self-conscious, and incompatible with the other moms. The way out was talking ... and listening. The more I opened up, the more I realized that many other moms (and dads) had similar feelings of inadequacy, but also that often we are much harsher judges of ourselves than anyone else is. In the long run, confidence came from following my instincts as a parent.

Vita, mother of George

The "good enough" mother

Freeing yourself from Supermom's tight grip is about moving toward self-acceptance as a "good enough" mother. Instead of wishing you were a goddess, think of yourself as a gardener. This is a lovely way to understand psychoanalyst Donald Winnicott's "good enough" mom—who nourishes and sustains her baby with love and gentle, attentive care. Through containing strong feelings, she offers a secure base.

However, the good enough mother isn't limitless or a saint. She feels the emotional push–pull both toward and away from her baby. She feels conflicted and sometimes she makes mistakes. She is human. Even the most attuned mothers get it "right"—by tuning in and responding sensitively to meet their baby's needs—only around a third of the time. What is most important is a good enough repair.

First, this is about noticing your own thoughts and feelings and self-soothing (*see p126*). Then you can reconnect with your baby through cuddles and soft words. The repair teaches them that something positive can come out of a difficult moment or a tough day. So have "good enough" as your benchmark, and mindfully let yourself off the hook of perfect parenting.

Gratitude Jar

Consumer culture bombards us with reminders of how, as mothers, we should be doing more, better. Practicing gratitude is an antidote to all the striving, helping you to cope.

1

Jot down three things each day that you feel grateful for—ideally before bed as cultivating gratitude is known to enhance sleep. Write notes on pieces of paper and then pop them into your gratitude jar.

2

Try not to repeat the same things, and be specific. For example, write "enjoying breakfast" and "appreciating the woman who smiled at me." Include small wins, such as "finishing a hot drink."

3

If you wish, extend gratitude to your partner and those in your support circles.

4

Now shift your focus of appreciation to you and your baby. What small yet significant acts of love might your baby feel grateful to you for today? Consider cuddles, talking, and singing to your baby—all those little things that help them feel safe.

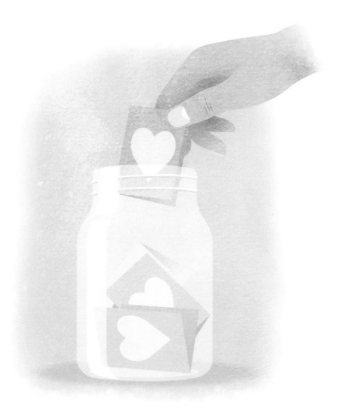

5

If you find it hard to keep it up, create a phone reminder or put post-it notes on the fridge to prompt you.

6

If you prefer, keep a gratitude diary. By noting what you're grateful for and what lifts your mood, you're rewiring neural brain pathways to focus on appreciation and contentment.

Meditative Stroll in Nature

On the days when you have more energy or need space, take your baby outside for a mindful walk. Tune in to your senses to stay anchored with this calming grounding technique.

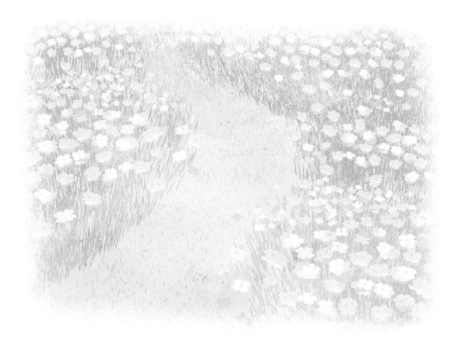

1

Take a few deep breaths. Bring mindful attention to your senses. Start by looking up and around you.

2

Name **five** things you can see. They can be close by or further away, such as your stroller, flowers, people, or clouds. Your baby can't see in color yet, but as they grow, practice seeing the world through their eyes.

3

Name **four** things you can hear. Tune in to sounds nearby, such as birds singing or people talking. Listen without judgment. Become aware of distant sounds, such as the low hum of traffic.

4

Name **three** things you can touch. Notice the textures and sensations. For example, the feel of the soft grass.

5

Name **two** things you can smell. Mindfully inhale the scent of something, such as your baby's neck, a grounding oil you carry with you, or the fresh air.

6

Name **one** thing you can taste. This could be your drink, or bring to mind a favorite thing you'd love to taste. Practice this simple, effective exercise whenever you're out and about with your baby.

Nourishing Herbal Teas

Staying hydrated can be a challenge when you're feeding and caring for your baby. Enjoying an herbal tea is a refreshing wellness ritual as well as being a good source of hydration.

Listen to your body's signals and respond mindfully when you feel thirsty. Make sure you're drinking enough fluids, particularly if you're breastfeeding. Given their health properties, herbal teas are a good choice for new moms, when enjoyed in moderation—have just one or two cups of weak tea a day. Herbs considered healthy and safe for new mothers include **nettle**, **chamomile**, **oat straw**, **rose hip** (*see right*), **red raspberry leaf**, and **lemon balm**. Chamomile and lemon balm teas are wonderfully calming options that aid digestion. To boost energy, opt for rose hip and nettle tea, which is rich in minerals and vitamin C.

"Mindfully making and enjoying your herbal tea is a small but important act of self-care."

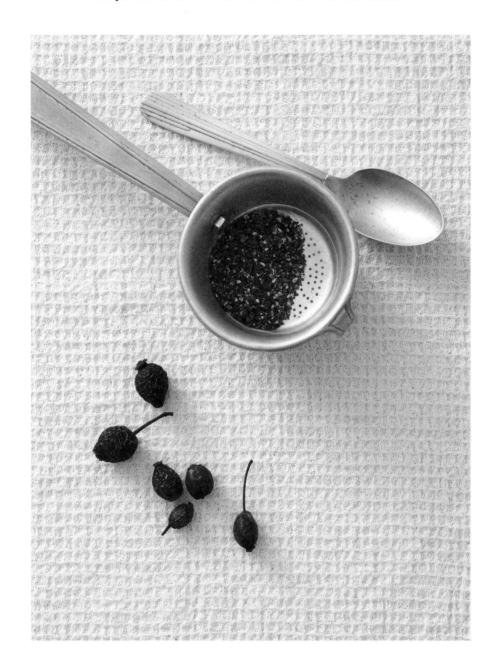

Meditative Scar Massage

After a Cesarean, you may have mixed feelings about your incision. Combining massage with mindful breathing is a powerful healing ritual, helping you connect to your postpartum body through gentle touch.

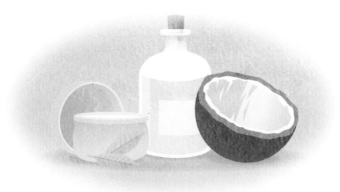

1

You can begin Cesarean scar massage as soon as your wound is fully dry and healed, usually after six to eight weeks. When you feel ready, check with your doctor or midwife.

2

Lie down and place your hand on your stomach. Breathe with purpose into your diaphragm. Move your hand gently on or just above your scar.

"Gentle abdominal massage helps to reunite brain and body, promoting blood circulation and healing."

3

Rub a little oil in your hands and start by massaging in large clockwise circles all over your abdomen. Use natural cold-pressed oils rather than synthetic oils. Good options include vitamin E oil, coconut oil, and rose hip oil.

4

If you're reluctant to touch your scar directly, try sweeping a cotton ball softly over it.

5

When ready, place your fingers just above your scar and gently push down, moving your fingers up and down and from side to side. You shouldn't feel any pain, but it may feel tender. If you feel any areas of restriction, gently push the tissues until you feel them release.

6

Try one minute of massage a day, building up to five minutes. Each time, say, "My body is wonderful—touch will help it heal."

Eating Regularly for Energy

When you're exhausted, it's tempting to reach for a package of cookies for a quick energy boost, but after a sugar rush, the crash will leave you feeling even worse. Graze on nutritious, healthy snacks instead.

Skipping meals causes your blood sugar to drop, leaving you depleted in energy and more vulnerable to anxiety and feeling overwhelmed. Eating regularly and choosing the right foods is vital for sustaining energy levels—a must for all new moms. If you're breastfeeding, you're likely to want to snack more to maintain energy levels. Have a bowl of mixed, unsalted **nuts** and **seeds** or **fruit** handy in your "zen zone" (*see p86*) to graze on while feeding.

For an easy protein-rich snack, hard-boil a batch of eggs. **Hummus** (*see right*) with slices of **carrots**, **cucumber**, **peppers**, and **celery** are good, healthy options. Combine with bowls of nutritious low glycemic index (GI) fruit such as **blueberries**, **strawberries**, and **pears**. If you tire of hummus, try **oat cakes** with **cashew butter** and sliced **banana** to tide you over.

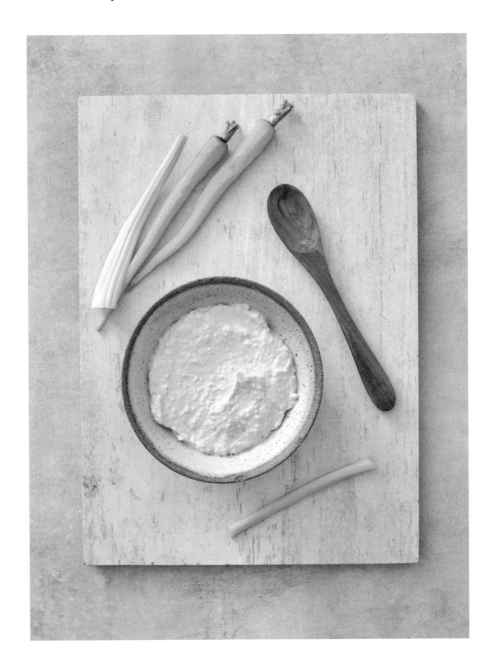

Connecting to Music

For centuries, music has been used as a powerful tool. Known for its therapeutic effects, mindfully listening to music allows mutual soothing with your baby, as well as helping you reconnect to your prebaby self.

Amid the mothering merry-go-round of feeding and changing, the prebaby you can feel far away. What about the you who loves feeling free and dancing into the early hours? Listening to much-loved tracks from different stages of life can help you reconnect to parts of your identity that feel so dim and distant right now. Just one uplifting song associated with happy memories can powerfully boost your mood. It's also a helpful reminder that the lighter part of you *is* in there somewhere. Even if it has temporarily slipped from view.

"*Let music be your therapy—whether you switch on the radio or stream your favorite tracks.*"

MINDFULLY LISTENING TO MUSIC

Music has been shown to reduce anxiety, depression, and fatigue; lift mood; and improve responses to pain. Really focus attention on the tempo and different layers in the music.

Select your songs

Create specific playlists to help you manage certain times of day. For example, choose a selection of up-regulating songs to energize you and your baby. In the evening, listen to a down-regulating playlist to unwind before bed or soothe your baby.

Creating musical memories

Whether you listen to classical, dance, rock, or reggae, get your baby actively involved. We know babies form musical memories as early as in utero, showing a preference for songs played to them in the womb one year after birth.

Energizing music

Just as it does for you, music helps regulate your baby's emotional states. Infants are most stimulated by fast-paced music that mimics their heart rates—so crank up the volume and create the kitchen disco vibe. Babies delight in repetition so keep playing much-loved songs to them. Enjoy dancing together!

Calming music

Singing or playing a lullaby is used universally to soothe and signal sleep time. Slow-paced music, with free movement and minimal change, switches off pain receptors in our brains to prepare us for sleep. As you sing, sway and rock your baby—they love the rhythmic regularity in both sound and movement.

Shrinking Down Your Inner Critic

Pressure to parent perfectly assails us—inside and out, on- and offline. Get to know your inner critic, noticing what it says and the feelings behind it. Then take compassionate action to disempower this mean bully.

1

Bring to mind a stressful time when you berated yourself—perhaps a situation that left you feeling inadequate as a mom.

2

Imagine your inner critic as external to you. If your inner critic vanished, you might feel relieved. But notice any fears about letting go of it, for example, becoming neglectful.

3

Imagine what happens when your inner critic runs the show. You might see it as a critical parent or nagging voice. Tune in to what your critic said to you in that stressful moment.

4

Reflect on how this savage bully left you feeling. Did you feel punished and shamed? Did you think "I'm a failure"?

5

You may notice that your inner critic isn't caring or supportive. What hurt feelings lie behind it, signaling an unmet need?

6

Make a mindful choice to connect to your compassionate self. How does your kind, committed, wise self show you understanding that mothering is hard and that all parents struggle? Use the affirmations below to help you shrink down your inner critic.

Tell yourself gently:

"There's no right way to mother."

"I'll try going with the flow."

"It's okay to mess up—I'm learning.
I'm doing the best I can."

"Tomorrow is a new day—
I'll start afresh then."

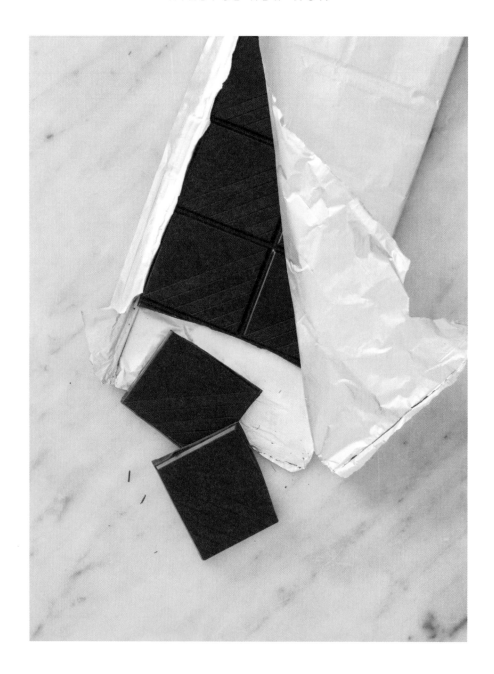

Mood-boosting Foods

In the emotional ups and downs of early motherhood, making mindful choices to eat feel-good foods rich in tryptophan and magnesium can positively impact your mood and well-being.

Tryptophan is an essential amino acid that helps your body produce niacin, which plays a key role in creating the neurotransmitter serotonin. Serotonin is associated with well-being and happiness, regulating anxiety and mood and reducing depression. **Chicken, turkey, eggs, cheese, fish, tofu,** and **milk** are all good sources of tryptophan. It is also found in **peanuts, pumpkin seeds,** and **sesame seeds**, so snack on these and sprinkle over salads for a healthy lunch.

Magnesium is crucial for mood and energy. Reduced levels can leave you feeling tired, tense, and agitated and can affect concentration, memory, and quality of sleep (*see also p160*). To boost your intake, eat plenty of **avocados, tofu, whole grains,** and **legumes.** Add **cashews, almonds,** and **Brazil nuts** to your snack bowl, and treat yourself to **dark chocolate** with at least 70 percent cocoa content (*see left*) for maximum benefit.

Managing Judgment

As a new mom, managing the endless stream of advice from relatives, friends, and strangers can be exhausting. To help you respond rather than react, cultivate "fierce compassion" by drawing clear boundaries.

1

You may notice feeling intensely raw and vulnerable in the fourth trimester—and advice, however well meaning, can easily be received as criticism. Call on the counsel of your trusted inner circle when required. And remember, you are the expert of you and your baby.

2

To deal with unwanted advice, take a few deep, conscious breaths to create space, allowing you to step back.

3

If the advice feels attacking or a threat to the way you are choosing to mother, acknowledge any difficult feelings. Rest a hand on your heart to show them compassion.

4

Tune in to any thoughts circling. If it feels important to validate your choice, do so. Otherwise, ask yourself: "Does this deserve my energy?"

Consider these verbal
responses to advice if one feels
necessary. Smile and say:

"Thank you, I'll bear that in mind."

"My doctor said X, I'm following their
advice on that."

"Thanks, I appreciate your thoughts.
There are many ways to parent;
this is the approach I feel
happy with."

5

If you feel overwhelmed, redirect your attention to your
feet. Becoming aware of the soles of your feet connected to
the earth is grounding. This simple act will help you feel
calmer, allowing you to process the comments with less
judgment. Hold onto what feels valid and let go of the rest.

Grounding Essential Oils

Many moms feel a sense of dread as the "witching hour" approaches, when babies become fractious. Use essential oils to ground yourself amid these turbulent storms.

You may find that your otherwise content baby comes undone toward the end of the day. Meanwhile, you are exhausted and your head feels very full. To restore a sense of calm, place one or two drops of your chosen essential oil on a cotton wool ball or handkerchief and inhale the scent. **Lavender**, **patchouli**, and **rose geranium** are all recommended for bringing stillness and balance. **Neroli** is similarly grounding, and **Roman chamomile** (*see right*) is beautifully soothing for both you and your baby. Just remember less is more with essential oils—you don't need much for a powerful effect.

"You may find that as your breath and heart rate slow, your baby picks up on your calmer state."

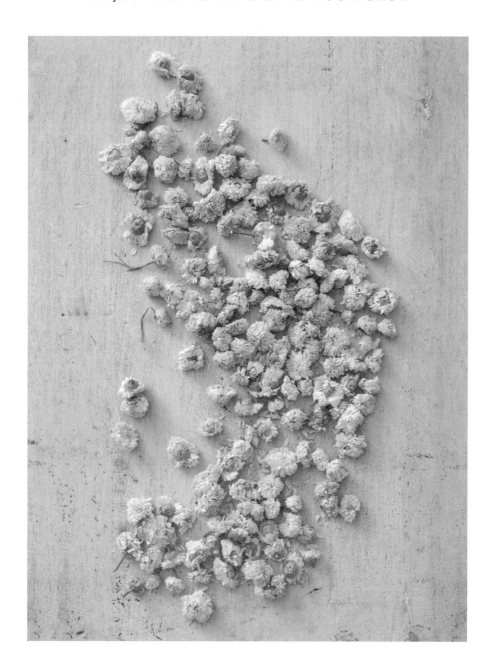

Your Special Place

Being a new parent may feel overwhelming at times—having a "special place" to go to in your mind shrinks down anxiety. Recalling happy memories can be an effective way to self-soothe and find calm.

1

Tune in to your natural rhythm of breath. Bring to mind your special calming place—this could be a sandy beach, a forest, or a garden bench.

2

Take a look around: what do you see? A shimmering blue sea or vibrant green meadow? Now focus on what you can feel, maybe the warmth of the sun or a gentle breeze. Are you aware of any smells? Perhaps salty sea air or freshly cut grass. What sounds do you notice? The gentle lapping of waves or birds singing?

3

Imagine that your special place feels joy simply in you being there. Smile softly and relax.

4

Now imagine inviting a compassionate "other" into your special place. This can be a nurturing figure, animal, image, color, or natural form. Whatever you choose will be your perfect nurturer in every way—radiating qualities such as understanding and warmth.

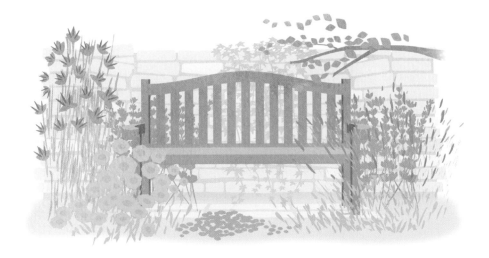

5

Consider what wisdom your
nurturer could offer you. It
might tell you: "It's going to
be okay. You are loved.
I'm here with you."

6

Notice any relaxed and
pleasant sensations in your
body as you call to mind
your loving guide in your
safe sanctum.

7

Consider what one word you
could associate with your
calm place. Hold that word in
your mind alongside those
relaxed feelings.

8

Take these peaceful feelings
with you for the rest of the day.
When a storm comes, call on
them and your word to help
you feel soothed and safe.

Reflecting on Motherhood

Figuring out what kind of mother you want to be will help you choose what advice is meaningful and what to disregard. Let your values guide your mothering style—making wise choices that fit best with your family.

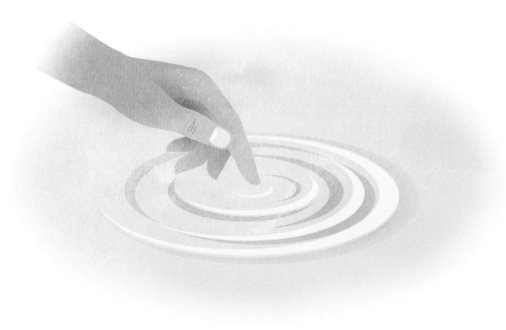

1

Sit somewhere quiet where you can think for a moment. Jot down some notes as you complete this reflective exercise.

2

Imagine that your baby is grown up. Consider what they might look like and what they may be doing.

3

What are your hopes for your grown-up child? What qualities and attributes would you hope to have encouraged in them?

4

Now imagine you can hear your child, all grown up, talking to a friend about how lucky they are to have a mom like you. What, specifically, do they appreciate most about you? What might they say is special about you?

5

Come back to you and your baby now. If you could mother exactly the way you wanted— free of external judgment and your inner critic—what would you do differently?

6

When you've finished, review your notes. Summarize any key values on paper. Read these whenever you feel unsure about a decision or challenge, and let your values guide you.

Practice and Posture

When you're sleep-deprived and focused on your new baby, it's hard to imagine having time to exercise. But creating a space to come back to your body after birth is a wonderful way to reconnect to yourself again.

Caring for your baby can leave you feeling physically worn out. Taking time to release the tension in your shoulders helps relieve aches and pains as well as recenters you emotionally. As a new mom, it is recommended that you don't return to exercise until six weeks after a vaginal birth and 12 weeks post–Cesarean section. Before returning to a regular yoga practice, your midwife, yoga teacher, or physician should check your core abdominal muscles for separation. When ready to begin, approach this yoga sequence slowly and gently with awareness of how you're feeling in your body.

"These gentle postures will help relieve tension from the demands of tending to a newborn."

20-MINUTE SEQUENCE

Gentle yoga postures will help you regain trust in your body, supporting a kinder relationship with it. Start slowly and gently by doing several of the poses, and as you regain your energy and strength, build up to the full sequence.

01

KNEES TO CHEST

Lie on your back, resting your head on a pillow. Draw your knees into your chest, one at a time. Bring your hands around your knees and gently hug them in toward your chest. Rock for a minute or two, feeling a lovely massage of your lower back. Make the movements as large or small, fast or slow as feels comfortable. To finish, roll onto your side and carefully push up to seating.

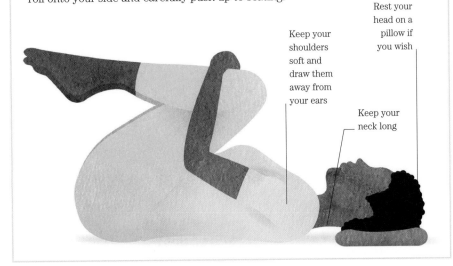

Keep your shoulders soft and draw them away from your ears

Rest your head on a pillow if you wish

Keep your neck long

02

SEATED EAGLE POSE

Sit comfortably, spine upright, and stretch your arms wide. Hug yourself, bringing your left elbow and arm above your right arm. Keep your elbows crossed over and lift both arms and hands toward the sky. Allow your wrists to circle around each other so your palms touch, your arms intertwined. Breathe comfortably. As you exhale, draw your shoulders softly down and lift your elbows away from your chest. Hold for 10 breaths, then bring your arms down and repeat with your right arm on top.

Draw your elbows up toward the sky

Keep your shoulders pulled down

Maintain an upright spine throughout

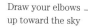

03

CAT

Move slowly onto your hands and knees into Tabletop. Your hands should be directly under your shoulders, your knees hip-width apart, your back flat. Breathe comfortably. As you exhale, move your spine into an arch shape, drawing your back up toward the sky. Hold, then press through your hands as you release your shoulders away from your ears. If you can, softly push your spine up a little more and hold for 5–7 breaths. Gently engage your pelvic floor, but only if it feels comfortable. Return to Tabletop and repeat three times.

RELEASING TENSION

In this lovely grounding pose, mindfully focus on your breath to release any tightness or tension.

Pull your shoulders down away from your ears

Arch your back like a cat

Push your hands into the floor to ground you

04

TABLETOP WITH CALF STRETCHES

From Tabletop, press your hands into the floor and find a steady position. Stretch one leg back, tuck your toes under, and extend through your heel. Breathe in and, as you exhale, lengthen down the back of your leg for a lovely calf muscle stretch. Hold for up to 10 breaths if comfortable. Return to Tabletop, then repeat with the other leg. Repeat if you wish, then push back to kneeling and carefully stand up.

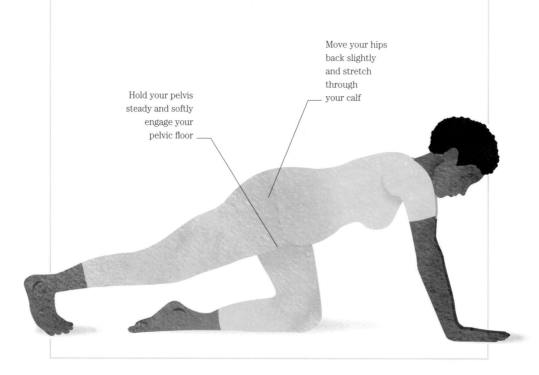

Move your hips back slightly and stretch through your calf

Hold your pelvis steady and softly engage your pelvic floor

05

MOUNTAIN POSE

Stand with your feet hip-width apart. Softly engage your legs, drawing your inner arches and knees upward so you feel stable and grounded. Engage your pelvic floor muscles to help with stability. Lengthen your spine and neck. Become aware of the gentle movement of your breath in the upper body, creating a sense of lightness, expansion, and ease. Hold for around a minute.

Draw the crown of your head upward

Lengthen your spine in both directions

Softly engage your lower stomach muscles

Spread your feet out to ground you

06

SEATED FORWARD FOLD

Sit comfortably on a block or cushion and stretch your legs straight out in front of you. Bend your knees a little if more comfortable. Stretch your arms up toward the sky, lifting out of your pelvis to create as much length as you can. Softly fold forward, letting your hands rest alongside your legs. Don't push or pull into this pose, just allow yourself to be and tune in to your breath. Feel the gentle rhythm of it come and go. Hold for up to 10 breaths.

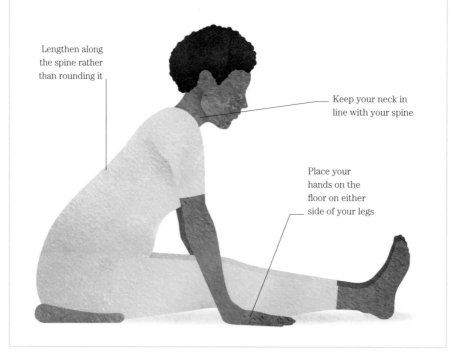

Lengthen along the spine rather than rounding it

Keep your neck in line with your spine

Place your hands on the floor on either side of your legs

07

SIDE-LYING RESTORATIVE POSE

Lie down on your side, placing a cushion under your head to support your neck. Bend one or both knees, placing cushions or blocks between them, resting them slightly in front of you on the ground. Let your lower arm softly rest on the floor in line with your shoulder nearest the ground. Allow your upper arm to rest wherever feels comfortable. Breathe, soften, and simply let go. Hold for as long as you wish.

FEEDING YOUR BABY

This pose is very relaxing and is a wonderfully restful position in which to feed your baby.

Close your eyes to allow you to fully rest

Use cushions or blocks for comfort

Focus on your breath

"Give yourself permission to just be, focusing on your breath."

REEMERGING WITH YOUR BABY

From three to six months, you may be settling into your role and enjoying lots of smiles. To help you cope with sleep deprivation, draw on compassionate meditations and visualizations, natural remedies, and nutritional advice targeting mood and sleep. Practice mindful speaking and listening to connect with your partner or co-parent.

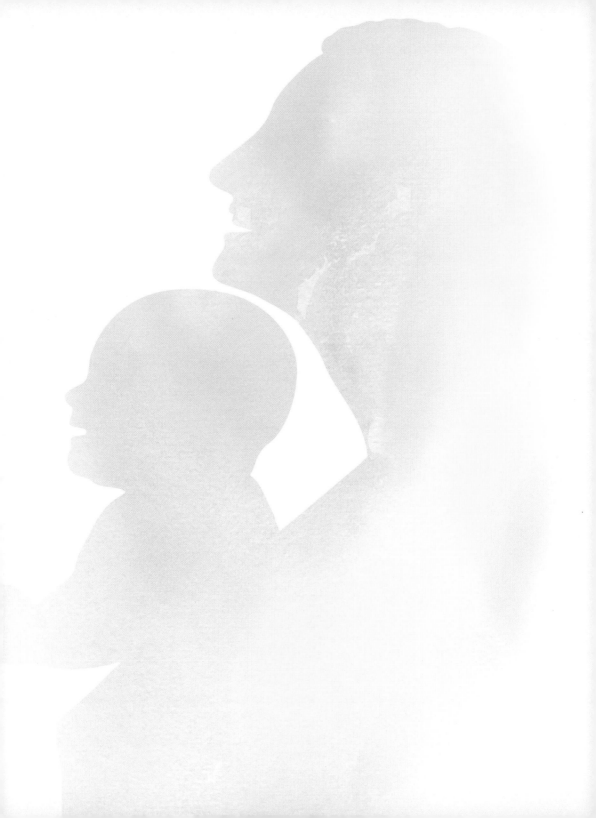

Reemerging with Your Baby

As your little one becomes more interactive, rewarding you with squeals and smiles, your heart can feel ready to burst. Celebrate sparkling moments of connection— they show how far you and your baby have come.

As your baby moves out of the newborn stage, you may feel a sense of emerging from your baby bubble to connect with the world again. You may be getting out more, meeting other moms for lunch, and going to parent and baby groups. You may also be finding more of a rhythm with your baby, or at least learning some of their feeding and sleeping patterns.

Take time simply to be with your baby, turn-taking, and mirroring their actions. They love it when you respond to their babbling with words, and these playful interactions help build their self-esteem and are a key part of your baby's development (*see p152*). Continue to take mindful walks with your baby (*see p116*), pointing out the things you can see, hear, or smell. Now that your baby is awake for longer periods, you may notice new challenges. One of which is, very likely, coping with cumulative exhaustion from all the broken sleep. While babies become more alert and sleep less during the day, most will continue to wake for food and comfort at night for a while yet. Use natural remedies to help enhance your sleep (*see p164*) and yoga to reenergize or restore you as needed (*see p174*).

Sleep deprivation

As a new mother, it can feel like you're walking a tightrope. Some days, when you've slept well, you feel invincible, juggling tasks with the agility of an acrobat. Other days, after nights of snatched sleep, you can feel raw, vulnerable, and full of despair. Sleeping in one- to two-hour blocks deprives you of both deep and REM sleep, important for dreams, learning, and memory. New mothers describe a tiredness so heavy that they find themselves putting house keys in the fridge and googling whether a woman can die from lack of sleep.

Difficult thoughts and feelings

Sleep deprivation is no joke—the mounting sleep debt causes physical exhaustion, reduced energy, irritability, short-term memory loss, and difficulty concentrating. In addition, chronic sleep disturbance is associated with depression and anxiety. You may feel so tired that you worry your baby might inadvertently come to harm. These fears are little talked about yet incredibly common. Studies show nearly every single woman experiences unwanted, intrusive thoughts of accidental harm coming to her baby. One in two women also report intrusive thoughts of intentionally harming their baby—even though they would never deliberately hurt their child. Given their taboo nature, these tormenting and upsetting thoughts usually evoke

»

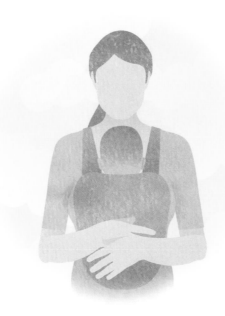

149

intense shame, horror, guilt, and a lack of control. Many women interpret these vivid visions as a sign that they're a bad mom. However, the very fact moms feel ashamed or horrified about having these thoughts is a strong sign that they're not going to hurt their baby.

Mindfulness allows you to step back from unpleasant intrusions, without getting hooked by them and judging yourself a bad mom for having had the thought (*see p172*). However, intention is key. If you find yourself having an overwhelming desire or intention to hurt yourself or your baby, please seek help urgently (*see p214*).

Coping with lack of sleep

A cruel trick of sleep deprivation is the way it distorts our perception of our ability to cope. Being woken multiple times in the night is understandably stressful. Breastfeeding mothers can experience nursing aversion and feel "touched out"—and may be consumed with self-critical thoughts such as "I'm failing—I can't cope." These fear-based beliefs are partly shaped by the Supermom myth, dictating that perfect moms must always be able to soothe their baby. Paying attention to your emotions in the moment means turning toward and tending to your

66 99 A MOTHER'S STORY

Before the birth of my daughter, I knew about sleep deprivation, but I don't think anything can truly prepare you for it. After coming home, I managed to get only a few hours here and there. I was in a constant state of shock and survival mode, my dwindling energy spent on feeding and protecting my baby. I began having intrusive thoughts and was terrified that these

thoughts meant I was going mad, so I kept them to myself. Eventually, I learned that these kinds of thoughts are common and I felt seen. They became less dominant and I knew then there was nothing wrong with me. Once my anxiety levels settled, sleep finally came, and I could begin to enjoy the time with my baby.

Pippa, mother of Peggy

You may reflect on the impact of your 'ghosts in the nursery'— consider your angels, too."

feelings. Using your breath and body to find your internal place of safety allows you to access empathy and see the bigger picture, both for you and your baby. Use the grounding exercises on pages 168 and 170 to help you.

What you're able to tolerate depends on your own unique circumstances and early experiences. When you become a mother, the "ghosts in the nursery" can intrude. These "ghosts" relate to your own relationships with your primary caregivers, which teach you about yourself, others, and the world around you. If you weren't supported to feel soothed and safe as a child, the process of separating from your own baby, for example, to settle them to sleep, can stir up painful feelings. Creating space to share difficult feelings with your partner or a supportive other can be validating and containing, helping you feel more connected (*see p166*).

Looking after yourself

The emotional storms of the early months, heightened by sleep deprivation and pressure to parent perfectly, can result in you bouncing back and forth between "threat" and "doing" mode. When you're worn out and stressed, it's hard to find clarity or compassion for yourself or your baby.

A challenge for all mothers is learning to look after yourself as well as your baby. Activating your soothing system and being kind to yourself takes conscious effort—it won't just happen. Make mindful, compassionate choices, such as creating a calming bedtime routine (*see p164*) and choosing nutritious foods (*see p154* and *p160*). Try to make space for difficult emotions, recognize when your cup is overspilling, self-soothe, and prioritize "me time" by practicing yoga nidra (*see p158*) or restorative yoga (*see p174*).

Mindfully Appreciating Playtime

Play helps your baby understand the world as they learn to focus attention, take turns, and test new ideas. Their favorite plaything is you—try to relax and bring your mindful presence to these moments.

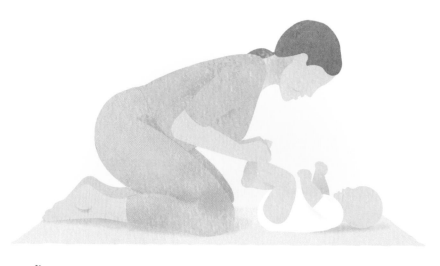

"*Play offers a wonderful insight into your baby's world.*"

1

Set aside 10 minutes of quality playtime a day to nourish your relationship with your baby. What your baby loves most is your attentive presence. Surrender to this special time.

2

Play offers a wonderful insight into your baby's world. It can also evoke anxiety or boredom, depending on your childhood experiences. Reflect on whether play was modeled to you and encouraged.

3

Resist pressure to teach your baby. They are discovering their ability to make an impact on the world. Notice any judgments or criticisms that arise and let them go. Simply observe and be curious.

4

Hold your baby to face you and mirror their facial expressions, noises, and actions. Babies love looking at human faces. Play peekaboo and lap games.

5

Watch your baby exploring different materials, textures, and shapes, such as a wooden spoon, a ball, or a stuffed animal.

6

As they play, try commentating. Narrate what you see—rather than intervening—as this gives voice to their experience.

7

Chat to your baby as they play. Over time, these conversations enrich language development.

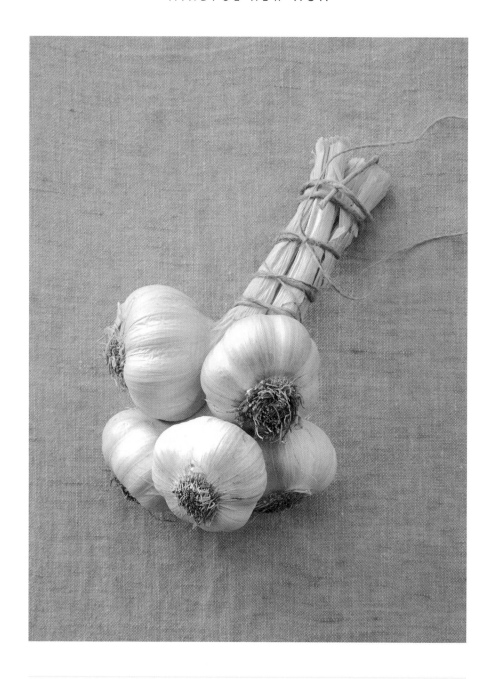

Prebiotics and Probiotics

Prebiotics and probiotics are essential for a healthy gut. As the fourth trimester can be an anxiety-provoking time, and evidence suggests some mood problems may be linked to gut health, aim to keep your gut in balance.

Prebiotics are nondigestible fibrous foods that feed the good bacteria; while probiotics increase the number of good bacteria in the gut. To boost your intake of prebiotics, include **onion, garlic** (*see left*), **leeks, asparagus**, and **chickpeas** in your meal planning. Probiotics are strains of live bacteria and yeasts (found in fermented foods) that can aid digestion, metabolism, and sleep. To increase your probiotic intake, eat more fermented foods, such as **kimchi, miso, kefir, sauerkraut, kombucha**, and **live yogurt**.

"Promising research has highlighted a link between maternal gut health and mood."

Mindful Speaking and Listening

Pregnancy and welcoming a new baby shifts dynamics in a couple's relationship. When so much energy is required to care for your little one, it may take conscious effort to reconnect with your partner.

This exercise invites you and your partner (or a supportive other) to create a safe, open space to truly listen to each other. Before you come together, consider what gets in the way of hearing each other. Feeling exhausted and stressed could lead to shutting down, or challenging and blaming the other, depending on your own reactivity style. Containing your baby leaves your head feeling full (*see p68*). To feel contained yourself, you may want empathetic listening—not problem-solving.

"*Parenting stress can lead to communication breakdown— create space to talk.*"

RECONNECTING WITH YOUR PARTNER

*Use this exercise as a reflective journey of discovery.
Discuss together first what you both hope to gain from
it, agreeing on the goal of shared understanding.*

Taking time to talk

Set aside 20 minutes weekly to ask the questions listed below. The first person responding shares their feelings honestly, without interruption or criticism. The second person then does the same.

Calm approach

Before answering each question, take several deep breaths. Check in with yourself, noticing any sensations, emotions, or thoughts. Ask yourself: "What is my intention here? What do I need?"

Importance of listening

While listening, offer your partner the gift of kind attention. Use your breath as an anchor to help you stay present. Bring a receptive attitude, returning to the breath whenever irritation or judgments arise.

Questions to ask

The first person asks each of the following questions in turn; the second person responds openly to them.

"How was your day?"

"How are you feeling?"

"Tell me one thing that has gone well this week."

"Tell me one thing that has felt difficult this week."

Solutions

When you've both responded, discuss possible solutions. If it's acknowledgment for what you're doing that is needed, ask for that. Or it may be a hug, or a logistical request, such as alternating your baby's bathtime. End by thanking each other for bringing an open presence.

Yoga Nidra

Yoga nidra is a state of consciousness between waking and sleeping, typically induced by a guided meditation. This powerful practice promotes rest and inner peace, offering profound restoration for exhausted mothers.

1

Lie down comfortably and allow your body to fully let go. Connect to your senses. Focus on each inhale and exhale. Feel each exhale soften the body.

2

State your heartfelt desire for how you would like to feel or be. For example: "I am enough." Imagine what it would be like if this was happening now.

3

Rotate attention around your body. Starting at your right thumb, mentally name each body part as you travel down the right side, then move to the left side.

4

Let your awareness soften each body part, then bring awareness to your breath. Observe your breath for 10 inhalations, silently repeating: "The body breathes in … the body breathes out."

5

Notice a sense of heaviness in the body. Now invite a sense of lightness in. Then alternate between the two sensations.

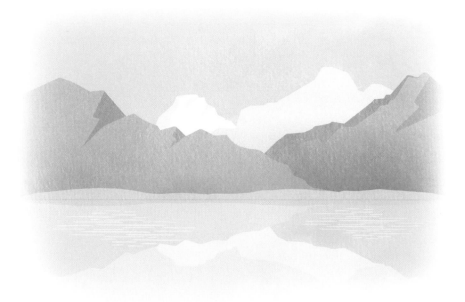

6

Imagine you're outside in nature, perhaps in your special place. Notice the surrounding beauty, tuning in to what you can see, hear, and smell. You feel relaxed and safe here. Breathe in the life-giving air. You can return to this place whenever you need to feel at peace and at ease.

7

Let awareness rest in your heart for a few minutes. Then begin to shift awareness from your inner to outer world. Reconnect to your physical body. Notice your breath, and slowly introduce movement back into the body. Offer yourself a moment of gratitude for gifting yourself this time to rest.

Sleep-enhancing Foods

Sleep deprivation can leave you feeling foggy with fatigue and unable to concentrate or fully enjoy your baby. To enhance sleep quality, focus on eating foods rich in melatonin, magnesium, and tryptophan.

To improve your sleep, try snacking on a few handfuls of **almonds** several hours before bed. Almonds contain melatonin, the sleep-regulating hormone, and magnesium. Magnesium is considered to have a sleep-enhancing property due to its ability to reduce levels of cortisol, which can interrupt your slumber. Evidence also suggests that moderate quantities of protein before bed may contribute to higher-quality sleep, so enjoy a **turkey** sandwich for your evening meal. Turkey is high in protein and contains the amino acid tryptophan, which enhances the production of melatonin. For a sleep-inducing drink, have two tablespoons of concentrated **tart cherry juice** (*see right*).

"Tart cherries are high in melatonin as well as tryptophan."

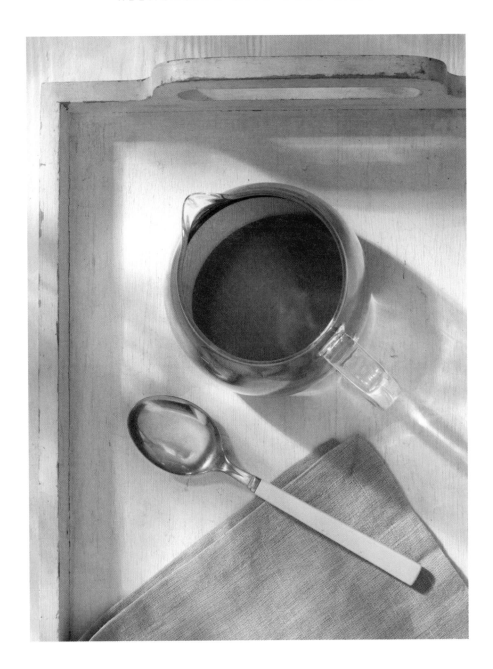

Leaves on a Stream

Remember, you are not your thoughts. Practice this exercise to separate yourself from your thoughts, feelings, and sensations. Notice and observe them without judging them or becoming hooked by them.

1

Sit comfortably. Use your breath to anchor you in the present moment. Imagine yourself sitting beside a gently flowing stream, with leaves drifting along the surface of the water.

2

Thoughts will come into your mind. With the next thought, place it on a leaf and allow it to float by. Do this with each thought, whether it's happy, sad, or neutral—place it on a leaf and let it glide by.

3

Let the stream flow at its own pace. Don't try to hurry it up or hasten your thoughts along. Simply allow them to come and go, without getting caught up in them.

4

If your mind tells you, "This is silly" or "I'm bored," notice those thoughts, place them on leaves, too, and watch them pass by.

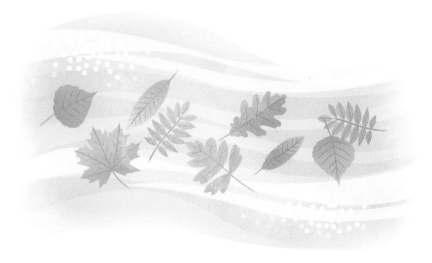

5

If an irksome or painful feeling arises, simply acknowledge it. Say inwardly, "I notice myself having a feeling of impatience or frustration" (or another troublesome feeling). Rest those thoughts on leaves and let them float by.

6

From time to time, you may get hooked by your thoughts. Acknowledge that this is normal.

7

If you do get distracted, as soon as you notice, gently redirect your attention back to the stream.

8

To finish, become aware of the ground beneath you and the air against your skin, slowly coming back into the room.

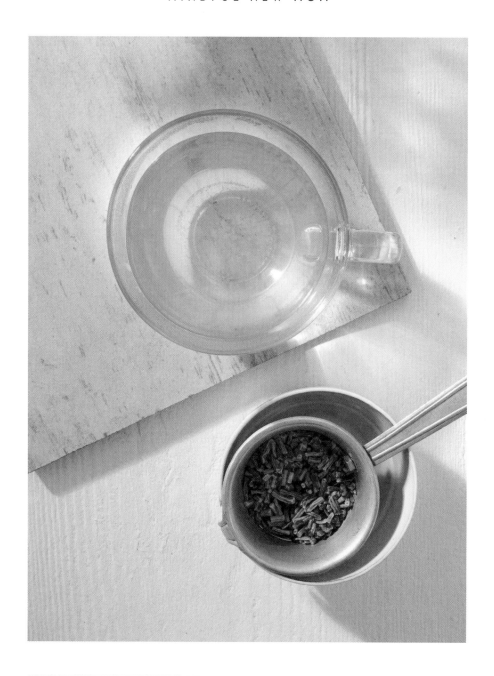

Calming Bedtime Rituals

After months of disrupted sleep, exhausted mothers may have to "relearn" how to sleep again. Create evening rituals, incorporating natural remedies such as calming essential oils and herbal teas, to help you unwind.

Carving out time for a bedtime routine isn't easy, but it will allow your mind and body to prepare for sleep. Make your bedroom a calm place: cool, quiet, and dark. Disengage from emotionally stimulating activities, such as social media or heavy discussions with your partner. Avoid eating a heavy meal or drinking alcohol for at least two hours before bed. Herbal tea is an ideal drink to have in the evening. One study of sleep-disturbed new mothers found that those who drank **chamomile tea** daily over two weeks reported better sleep. **Lavender tea** and **valerian tea** (*see left*) are also soothing and sleep-enhancing.

"Adding essential oils—Roman chamomile or lavender—to a warm bath also induces sleep."

Appreciative Inquiry

You bring your own stories to parenting as your personal history inevitably shapes your responses to your child. Together with your partner, bring conscious awareness to patterns you each learned growing up.

Experiencing a childhood in which either of you felt unseen, unheard, neglected, or maltreated can leave you disconnected from certain emotions. You may have learned ways of coping at the time to keep you safe, such as cutting off from particular emotions or attending more to the feelings of those looking after you than your own. One of you may have had a much happier upbringing than the other. Mutually sharing your experiences supports you both to bring awareness to any challenges and identify current emotional triggers that may stem from them.

"Together, recognize patterns you wish to reject or replicate to create your own scripts."

APPRECIATIVE INQUIRY AROUND PARENTING STYLES

Use this exercise to illuminate things from the past that you or your partner wish to leave behind, as well as positives that you both hope to take forward.

Supportive space

With your partner/co-parent, set up a kind, supportive space for these conversations (*see also p156*). Reflecting on past experiences may be triggering. Agree an intention to listen with respect and sensitivity. If differences arise, use your values to guide you.

A strengths-based approach

Discuss the nature of this appreciative inquiry. Instead of seeking to identify problems that need fixing, this approach appreciates that strengths, skills, and abilities reside in each other and your family unit. Listen for these.

Take time

Allow enough time to do this inquiry justice. The first person responding shares their feelings honestly, without interruption. You then alternate. Before either of you speak, focus on your breath, noticing any thoughts, feelings, or sensations.

The exercise

You (or your partner) begin by reflecting on aspects of the way you were parented that you appreciated and want to replicate as well as aspects you found challenging and want to do differently. The other person listens as an "ability spotter"—noticing all the strengths, attitudes, actions, values, or relationships that made the best outcomes possible. They then highlight these abilities by naming them. Then, repeat the exercise with the second person reflecting on their experiences of being parented (as above). End with a hug or holding hands.

Regulate, Reconnect, and Repair

Coping with crying can evoke intense feelings in any parent. Practice the three Rs—regulate, reconnect, and repair—to mindfully connect with yourself in challenging moments, before coming back to your baby.

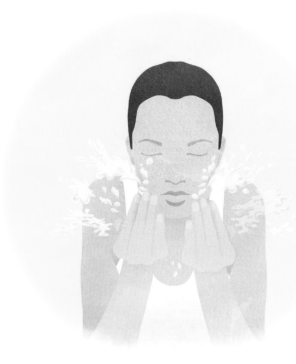

1

Your baby's cry is designed to elicit a strong reaction. Perceptions of your ability to cope are shaped by cultural ideas and your life experiences. You may fear being swallowed up by your baby's needs.

2

If you feel triggered, you need to find ways to come home to yourself first. Either put your baby down safely or hand them to someone else, and take time to regulate, reconnect, and repair.

3

Self-regulate. Splash your face with cold water. Notice any bodily sensations. Focus on breathing in for three counts and out steadily for six counts.

4

Reconnect with yourself. Tune in to your emotions and name them. For example: "I'm feeling tired/stressed/angry/fed up." Notice your inner critic: is it negatively comparing you to others or an idealized you? The antidote to shame is empathy—tell yourself gently: "It's okay to struggle—I'm human. Other moms struggle, too." After self-soothing, reconnect with your baby.

5

Repair with your baby. Cuddle them and help them understand their feelings. Say softly, "Crying is your way of communicating—I hear you. It's okay; Mommy's here."

6

Finally, find ways to soothe your baby that also soothe you. This could be gently swaying together or listening to relaxing music (*see p124*).

Healing Light

We develop different relationships with our emotions, depending on what was modeled to us growing up and in our culture. Externalizing our feelings, such as fear or anger, encourages understanding and acceptance.

1

Sit comfortably, allowing your mind and body to settle. Tune in to the in-flow and out-flow of your breath.

2

Call to mind a recent time when you felt moderately stressed—a situation that evoked feelings of anger, fear, shame, or sadness. Something difficult, but not traumatic, such as feeling angry after being woken by your baby and then shame for responding crossly.

3

Float back to that situation. Recall any words spoken and thoughts in your mind at the time. As you connect with the emotion attached to the most upsetting moments, bring your awareness into your body. Notice where in your body you feel the emotion most intensely with a kind curiosity.

4

Explore the emotion by imagining the sensations as a shape. Is the shape big or small? Abstract or clear? Rough or smooth?

5

As you breathe in, imagine your chest expanding to make room for the shape sensations. Now imagine breathing in a healing golden light. What happens to the shape sensations as your soothing healing light spreads out within you? Just be curious and notice.

6

As you make space for your shape sensations, notice what happens to it. Making room for a painful emotion doesn't mean liking it—just allow it to be there. Bring your caring presence to this emotion. When ready, slowly come back into the room.

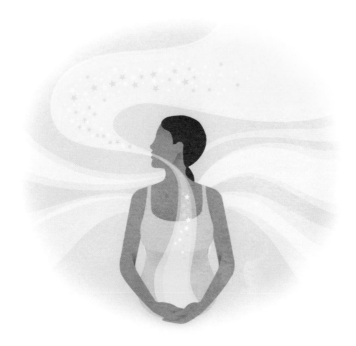

RAIN Meditation

Your baby is finally settled, yet sleep eludes you. Lying awake at night can unleash anxiety in your mind— magnifying future-focused worries and existential fears. Practice RAIN to recognize and nurture your worries.

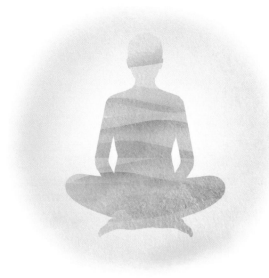

"Acknowledge and nurture painful feelings—they make you human."

1

Recognize

Simply naming the anxiety allows you to take an Observer position. Ask yourself, "What am I feeling inside me right now?"

Name it to tame it, such as, "I am feeling frightened."

Noticing and naming your emotions is the first step toward soothing your threat system.

2

Allow

Many mothers feel ashamed because they judge themselves as "bad" for even feeling or thinking a certain way. Bringing an open awareness and compassion to feared emotions helps shed the shame.

Acknowledge your feelings— try saying, "This is okay. Other moms feel like this, too."

3

Investigate

Move away from mental reactivity and come into your body. Ask yourself, "What am I fearing?" You may feel overwhelmed with fears of failure, unworthiness, or powerlessness. Or your fears may relate to worries about your baby's safety.

Where do you feel that fear in your body? Tune in to any stiffness or tension.

4

Nurture

After exploring your fear, ask yourself: "What does the hurt part of me need most?" Call on your compassionate self to offer you wise, kind words. Nurture your tricky brain for trying to keep you safe. Say tenderly, "Thanks, mind, for trying to protect me."

Observe any sense of freedom from painful thoughts and feelings.

Practice and Posture

Engaging in physical activity promotes recovery from giving birth. These gentle poses encourage you to shift your focus inward through breath awareness and reconnection to your body, helping boost energy.

Taking time to move your body and consciously connect to the breath will strengthen your muscles, increase flexibility, and help counter any stiffness. Inverted poses, such as Child's Pose and Legs Up the Wall, are wonderfully effective for nourishing your soothing system. These positions are beneficial both for your heart function and circulation and for balancing your energy. If anxious thoughts are preventing sleep, move into Legs Up the Wall. Daily practice of this inversion relaxes your mind and relieves pressure on your pelvic floor.

"Listen to your body. Use props for support and move at a pace that works for you."

20-MINUTE SEQUENCE

*Bring a nonjudgmental attitude to your practice. There's
no right or wrong in terms of what your body is capable of—
be gentle with yourself and let your body guide you as
you practice these regular, intentional movements.*

PELVIC FLOOR WORK

Lie on your back with your feet flat on the floor and
your knees bent. Relax your arms on the ground by
your body. Be aware of your breath expanding and
relaxing. On the exhale, softly engage your pelvic floor
muscles (front and back), drawing them in toward
each other and up to your heart center.
On the inhale, let them relax and release.
Repeat 10–20 times.

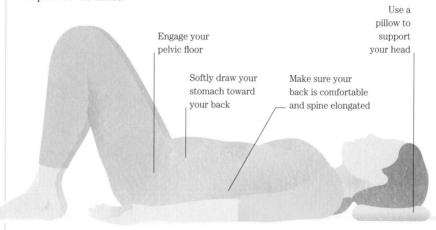

Engage your
pelvic floor

Use a
pillow to
support
your head

Softly draw your
stomach toward
your back

Make sure your
back is comfortable
and spine elongated

02

LEG STRETCH

Lie on your back with your feet flat on the floor and your knees bent. Hug one knee into your chest, place a strap around that foot, then extend your leg upward. Hold the strap lightly for support. Spread your foot and, on the exhale, encourage as much length through the back of your leg as is comfortable. Relax your back toward the ground, shoulders and jaw relaxed, neck long. Hold for 5–10 breaths, then repeat with the other leg.

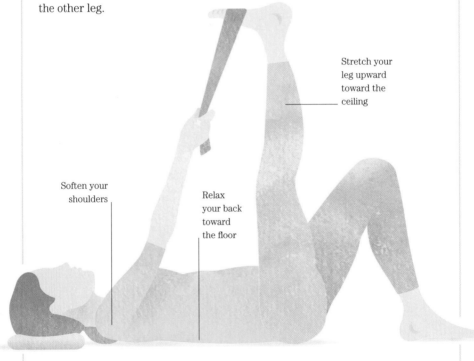

Stretch your leg upward toward the ceiling

Soften your shoulders

Relax your back toward the floor

03

LYING DOWN TWIST

Lie on your back and draw your knees up to your chest. Softly rock from side to side, enjoying the gentle massage on your back. Continue to draw both knees up toward your chest, then drop them over to the right. Breathe comfortably and allow your upper body to relax to the floor. Slowly stretch your arms out to the side, turning your head to the left. If more comfortable, relax your arms alongside your head. Hold for 5–10 breaths, then return to the rocking position and repeat on the other side.

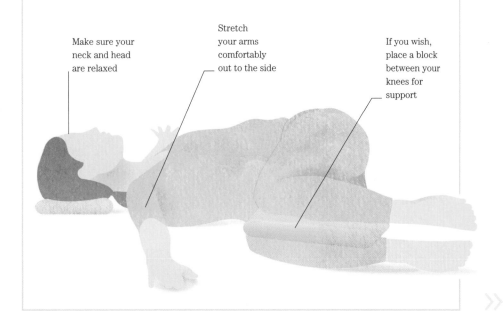

Make sure your neck and head are relaxed

Stretch your arms comfortably out to the side

If you wish, place a block between your knees for support

04

CHILD'S POSE

Carefully come into a kneeling position, adding support under your knees if needed. Softly allow your body to fold forward over your thighs. Bring your head to rest on a block. Rest your arms by your body, or bend them softly at the elbows, resting them in front of you. Breathe comfortably, feeling the breath in your back body expanding and releasing. On each exhale, draw your tailbone back and relax your shoulders away from each other. Hold for 2–3 minutes or longer if comfortable.

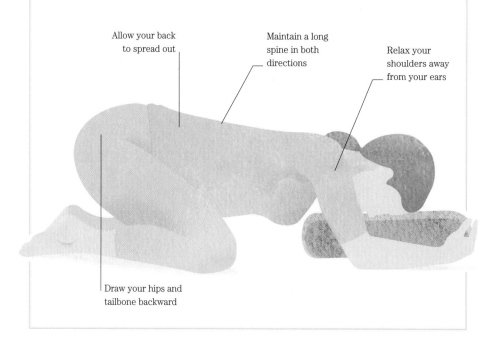

Allow your back to spread out

Maintain a long spine in both directions

Relax your shoulders away from your ears

Draw your hips and tailbone backward

05

DOWNWARD DOG

From Child's Pose, push up and back onto all fours. Spread your hands out, relaxing your head. On an exhale, tuck your toes under and softly lift your hips up, bringing your body into an upside-down V shape. Lift up onto your toes, knees softly bent. Focus on breathing comfortably, finding length in your upper body. When ready, carefully bend your knees to return to Child's Pose. Softly roll up and, using your arms to support you, push up to Mountain Pose.

UPPER BODY RELAXATION

This pose is great for reducing any tension, particularly in the shoulders and neck.

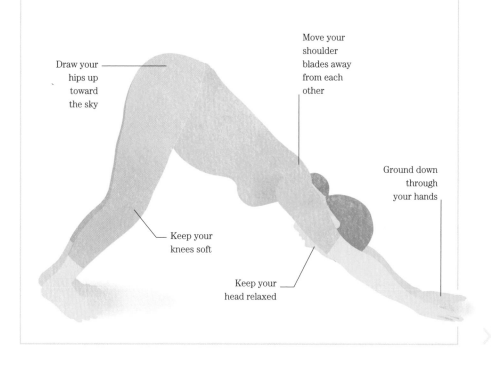

Draw your hips up toward the sky

Move your shoulder blades away from each other

Ground down through your hands

Keep your knees soft

Keep your head relaxed

06

STANDING FORWARD FOLD

From Mountain Pose, softly bend your knees and slowly fold your body forward from the hips. Keep both feet planted on the floor, knees slightly bent if you wish. Allow your upper body to hang forward, your arms dangling or touching the floor. Breathe comfortably, bending your knees as much as is needed for comfort. Allow the weight of your head to relax toward the pull of gravity and hold for 5–10 breaths, then return to Mountain Pose.

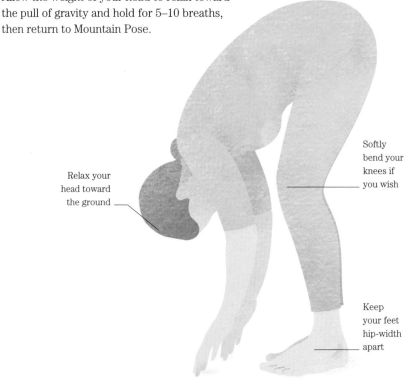

Relax your head toward the ground

Softly bend your knees if you wish

Keep your feet hip-width apart

07

LEGS UP THE WALL

Sit with your back against a wall, then swivel around and move onto your back, your bottom against or near the wall, your legs going up the wall. Rest your head on a cushion. Keep your lower back on the floor, even if this means being slightly away from the wall. Stretch your legs up to the sky. Bring your attention to your breath, inwardly saying, "I allow my body to slow down. Nothing matters but *this* moment ... and the next." Hold for up to 10 minutes.

AIDS SLEEP

This pose is very useful if you are stressed or unable to sleep.

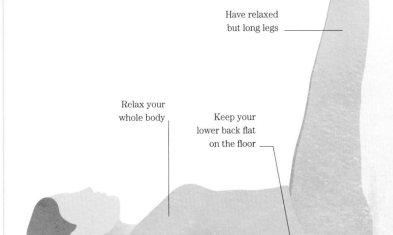

Have relaxed but long legs

Relax your whole body

Keep your lower back flat on the floor

CONNECTING THE DIFFERENT PARTS OF YOU

From six to 12 months, you may find more of a rhythm with your baby, but changes may also be ahead, such as returning to work (if you haven't already). Revisiting values, using compassionate visualizations, and prioritizing self-care can help you manage the process of separation and change, along with the mental load of parenting.

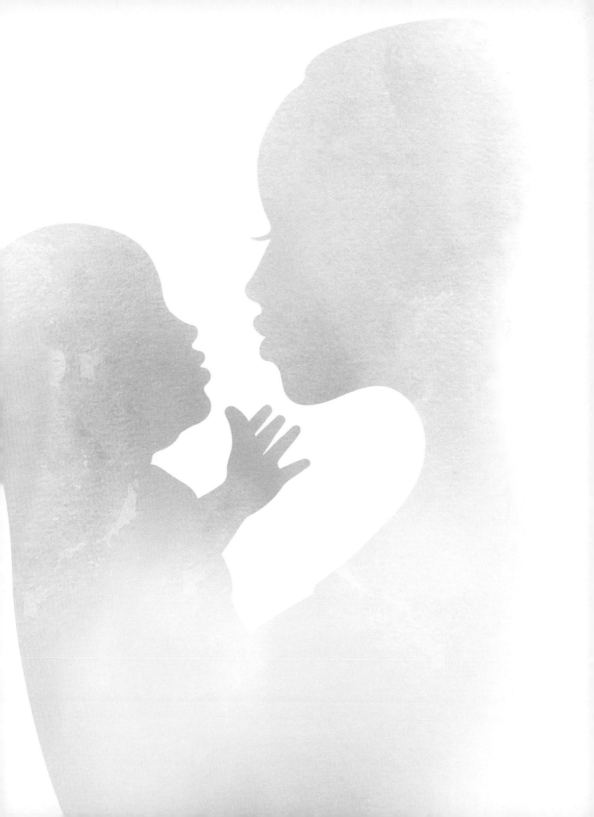

Connecting the Different Parts of You

Moving into the second half of your baby's first year, you may begin to grow in confidence as a mom. When your baby laughs, you'll want to bottle up those giggles—enjoy watching them explore their world with wonder.'

This period can be a time of moving toward reclaiming your sense of self, but this does not happen within a set time frame. Feeling more self-accepting and robust in yourself is in no way a fixed goal but rather a dynamic work in progress. As small pockets of time open up and you find more of a rhythm, you may reflect on important identity shifts during this life-changing transition. The all-consuming nature of the newborn phase required your time and energy in a way that may have felt overwhelming at times. Certain identities linked to your prebaby self were placed on pause. Now that your baby is becoming a little more independent, you may wish to begin reconnecting your old

"Learning your baby's unique cues and patterns is likely to make everyday things less stressful."

and new self. Returning to work and/or arranging childcare—whenever this happens for you—can present challenges in integrating multiple selves. This is normal—it takes time.

Appraising your values

What can help with reconnecting is returning to your values. Naming them supports this process (*see p40 and p136*), helping reconnect you with a sense of purpose and your preferred identity. You may wish to map out particular domains in which you live more or less in line with your values, such as relationships, work, health,

and leisure. If aspects of your prebaby self feel distant, consider realistic ways you can join those different parts. How can you reconnect with your preferred identities in a good-enough way? For example, if you identify as creative, could you write for 15 minutes a day? If health is a core value for you, find regular exercise that you enjoy.

Managing separation

Whether you are returning to work, you may find that unforgivingly high expectations imposed on you before having a baby no longer serve you. Having a new priority can bring

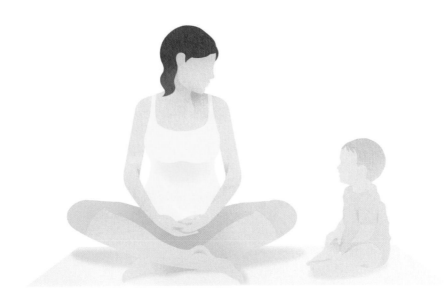

perspective and allow you to step back from any "all or nothing" beliefs based on old patterns of perfectionism. This encourages you to connect with yourself as a good-enough colleague and mother.

Learning to separate from your baby can, of course, feel anxiety-provoking initially. Visualizing goodbyes going well and finding a childcare arrangement you feel happy with will ease this transition (*see p200*). You may feel overjoyed to be going back to work or having time to yourself; you may be dreading the return; or you may feel a lot of conflicting feelings, including guilt, bringing discomfort in itself.

Remind yourself of the knapsack, so full and heavy with guilt and shame, that is gifted to each new mother after having a baby (*see p62*). Mindfully connecting with guilty feelings offers an opportunity to unpack your knapsack. How far is your guilt driven by impossible expectations of Supermom and your harsh inner critic? Try to realign those expectations (do they fit with your values?), and let go of cruel judgments. This will lighten your load.

The mighty mental load

Whether you work or not, bringing mindful awareness to the essential

---

❝❞ A MOTHER'S STORY

Going back to work was an opportunity for me to regain some of the balance I was used to—the balance of returning to a career and identity that I had spent most of my 20s fighting for and crafting. I knew I was good at my job. I wasn't sure I was good at being a mom all the time. What helped me was to know Eva was in good hands when I wasn't there. I had a good daycare and help from my mom and her dad. It really does take a village to raise a child, and it was the only way I could give myself 100 percent at work. I was excited the night before I went back, like the first day back at school. The fact that Eva slept through the night for the first time ever felt like a good omen.

Dami, mother of Eva

"Be conscious of how you expend your energy. Protect it as you would a precious jewel."

value of your mothering role is vital. This is partly about understanding your contribution in raising a new generation. Modeling skills of mindful compassion teaches your child emotional literacy, cultivating empathy and kindness and helping them thrive in life. Yet moms' responsibilities and strengths are often undervalued by society—and this can play out at home, too. Studies show that in heterosexual relationships, women overwhelmingly bear the domestic burden. One study showed that fewer than 7 percent of couples split the load. The mighty mental load falls heavily on women. This refers to taxing yet often overlooked tasks, from ordering groceries to arranging childcare.

What can help increase visibility of the mind-bending mental load is finding a language to address issues with your partner (*see p198*).

Taking care of yourself

Given that your job as a mother can feel unseen, yet perfection is expected, it's absolutely essential that you learn to soothe and contain yourself. This means bringing mindful awareness to your emotional capacity in any given moment, pausing to notice signs that your cup is about to spill over before you become overwhelmed.

In a society that puts a premium on productivity, rest really is rebellion. Claim time to connect to you. Schedule small acts of self-care, such as meditating for 10 minutes, playing music, or being in nature, to recharge and reset. Bigger things may be setting boundaries and gently saying "No." Prioritizing yourself will give you more headspace, allowing you to be the mother—and woman—*you* want to be. Honor your self-worth, complexity, and humanness in all its glory.

Compassionate Journaling

We often create stories of ourselves as "bad" mothers. Self-forgiveness through compassionate letter writing offers a way to recognize and release anger and blame linked to past regrets—moving you toward acceptance.

1

Take pen and paper and focus on your breath. Accessing your soothing system will support you to reflect in a kinder way.

2

Consider a situation or aspect of yourself that causes you to feel shame or not good enough. Note any thoughts and feelings, without judgment.

3

Next, imagine your compassionate self, calling to mind their qualities of strength and understanding. Feel soothed by their wise words and kindness.

4

Write a letter to yourself from this compassionate person. How would they encourage you to allow your painful feelings? How could they show that you are only human and all parents make mistakes?

5

As you write, reflect on feelings of shame and guilt arising from your painful situation. Shame is a feeling of "badness" about oneself, whereas guilt relates to behavior we fear might harm someone else.

6

Note that guilt feels heavy, but it can be constructive—leading you to recognize a difficulty you can repair. Write down what you could do differently next time. Perhaps pausing to self-regulate if stressed?

7

Write soothing words to let go of guilt: "In this moment, I forgive myself. Tomorrow I will start afresh."

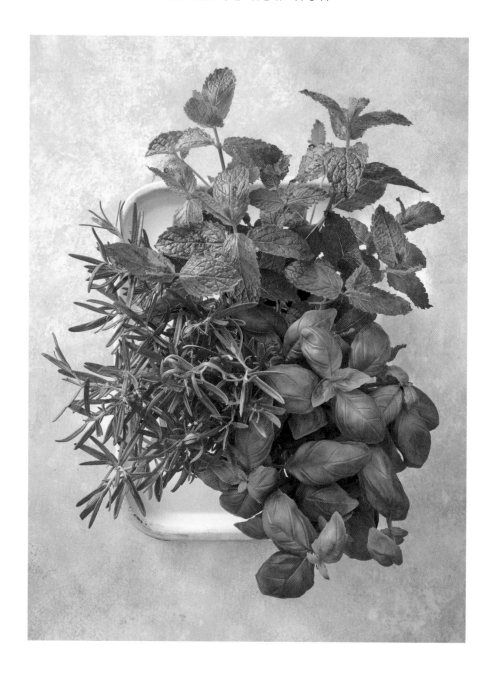

Mindful Meal Planning

For optimum health—plan, shop, and cook mindfully. Choosing pantry staples wisely and batch cooking will help with meal planning— saving you both time and energy.

Cooking is no fun when you're exhausted. Keep things simple and stock up on nutritious staples for throwing together quick, easy meals. Pantry essentials include canned **baked beans**, a great source of fiber; **tuna** in spring water for adding healthy goodness to salads; and **chopped tomatoes**, a tasty base for pasta and curry. Stock up on key herbs and spices, such as **basil**, **mint**, and **rosemary** (*see left*), as well as **cumin** and **cinnamon**, to inject flavor. Buy fresh soup packed with **beans**, **chicken**, or **lentils**, for easy energy-boosting lunches, and fill your freezer with high-quality, healthy meals.

Arrange a colorful assortment of fruits, such as **bananas**, **apples**, **kiwifruit**, and **satsumas** on your kitchen counter. Studies show that keeping fruit accessible makes you more likely to eat it. Jump-start your day with a smoothie: blend **blueberries**, **mango**, **ground flaxseed**, and **avocado**, topped off with water. For a more filling breakfast, add **banana**, **nut butter**, **almond milk**, and **oats** to a blender—whizz and enjoy!

Body Scan for Positive Body Image

Many new moms struggle with their body image. Cultivate a more accepting relationship with your postbaby body—mindfully extending respect and compassion to honor its efforts and achievements.

1

Lie down, legs uncrossed. Relax and tune in to your breath. Simply be with your body, without judgment.

2

Bring a kind, gentle attention to your legs and feet. With each exhale, allow any tension to melt away.

3

Focus on your pelvis and stomach, and appreciate their amazing work. Breathe in gratitude. Breathe out tension.

4

Notice any self-critical thoughts and allow kindness to wash them away.

5

Shift your attention to your chest. Become aware of your heart beating. Feel any sensations in your breasts. Breathe in compassion for this area. Breathe out tension.

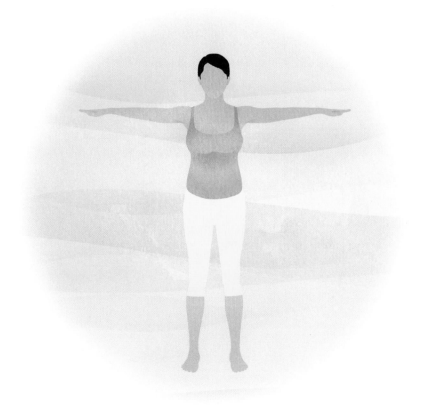

6

Move your focus to your back, shoulders, and neck. Feel them from the inside out. Invite loving care into your arms and hands for their soothing touch and strength. Breathe in thanks … breathe out tension.

7

Finally, appreciate your entire body. Say tenderly, "I respect my body. I honor and accept it, as it is."

Intimacy without Intercourse

Broken sleep and lack of opportunity and time can all impact intimacy after having a baby. Create ways to connect with your partner that don't involve intercourse to strengthen your relationship.

It is no secret that parents have less sex. The majority of new parents have concerns about changes to their sexual relationship, such as worries about when to resume sex after birth and, for moms, whether intercourse will be painful and how changes to their body image can impact sex postpartum. It takes most couples time to reconnect sexually. Feeling vulnerable, overwhelmed, or anticipating pain activates our threat system, blocking desire. You need to feel soothed and secure enough to be physically intimate. Create compassionate moments of connection—however fleeting—to bring you both closer.

"Use rituals of connection to show appreciation and stay attuned."

CREATING COMPASSIONATE CONNECTIONS

Whether it's a moment of eye contact or a meal out together, initiating and responding to bids for connection with your partner will help you both feel seen, valued, and loved.

Rituals of connection

Couples' therapist John Gottman suggests a daily six-second kiss (long enough to make it mindful!). Feel the sensation of your partner's mouth on yours and the brief bump of noses. Kissing releases oxytocin and dopamine and reduces cortisol. It's hard not to feel more loving after a kiss.

Intentional kindness

Show kindness in small, intentional ways. Enjoy breakfast together. Hold hands during a walk with the baby. Arrange a regular date night. Play cards, watch a favorite movie or TV show, or listen to much-loved music and dance together. Take the pressure off and keep expectations low.

Repair your relationship

Be aware when you're mind reading or expecting your partner to guess your wants and needs. Be forgiving of each other's limitations. When differences arise, self-soothe (*see p170*)—then reach out to repair.

Communication is key

Continue weekly, mindful check-ins with your partner (*see p156*). Create space to each share your thoughts and feelings about how parenthood has affected desire and intimacy. When you do feel ready, discuss possible adjustments, such as putting aside time to be intimate.

Relaxing Aromatherapy Massage

After holding your baby all day, you may long for physical contact that doesn't involve your child. Reconnect to the power of touch through aromatherapy massage, focusing on self-care rather than caregiving.

Just like your baby, you're soothed by touch, so enjoy some physical reconnection free of expectations. Suggest to your partner a mood-boosting massage using relaxing oils such as **lavender** (*see right*) or a citrus essential oil to reinvigorate you. Essential oils should always be diluted before being topically applied. For a restorative massage, use 3 percent dilution of your chosen essential oil to a carrier oil, such as **sesame oil**, **sweet almond oil**, or **jojoba oil**. This amounts to three drops of essential oil for every teaspoon of carrier oil.

"To make your own relaxing blend of essential oils, try combining ylang ylang, lavender, and bergamot."

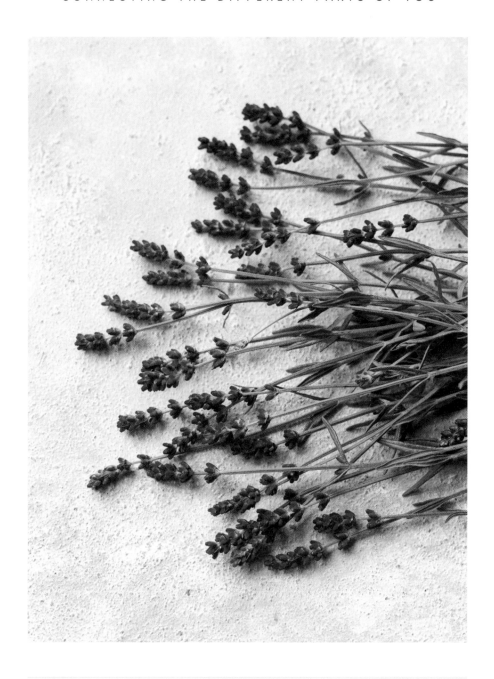

Sharing the Parenting Load

Supermom has us believe we should juggle it all—career, baby, homemaking, and the mighty mental load. The costs of this myth include exhaustion and burnout. Resist and recruit your partner to share the burden.

In interviews with both straight and same-sex, racially diverse couples, author Eve Rodsky heard a consistently expressed idea: men's time is valued far above that of women's time. Women also do the bulk of childcare. Tensions around work and household duties have significant consequences, prompting many women to opt out of the workforce. As a first step, you must both recognize that your time has equal value and that you each have different identities requiring time and emotional energy for you to flourish as people. Then you can work on rebalancing the mental and physical load of parenthood.

"Respect and factor equal time into your family timetable."

HOW TO SHARE
THE LOAD

Identify all the tasks that need doing, in line with your shared values. Cocreate a system—assigning who takes ownership of each task and responsibility for all steps involved.

Make time

There's never enough time. As a new parent, you become instantly interruptible, with myriad things competing for attention, not least your growing baby. All the while, you are monitoring all those invisible tasks that keep your home running smoothly. Set aside time to discuss your household workload.

Calculate the mental load

Cognitive work that keeps your mind forever churning ranges from meal prep and laundry cycles to arranging childcare. These under-the-radar tasks are often overlooked, even by the parent carrying them out, creating conflict. Together, name all the cognitive tasks that need doing, without assigning blame.

Define a system

Reflect on what you'd like to get out of discussions beforehand. Ask yourself, "What do I need—is it more support? More time for myself? A sense that we're a team?" Next, create a shared system to maximize productivity and redistribute the hours of domestic labor equitably.

Plan who does what

Map out all the tasks that need doing in a list or spreadsheet, specifying what's involved (anticipating needs, identifying options to fulfill those needs, decision-making, and monitoring progress). So if one partner does the weekly shopping, they take ownership for all steps involved, such as monitoring household essentials that need replenishing.

Managing Separation

Settling your baby in a new childcare setting and saying goodbye may feel heart-wrenching at first. Understanding it as a process that benefits you both, and visualizing it going well, can soften the separation.

1

Consider this transition as a normal developmental process relating to attachment. As a mother, you offer your baby a secure base. Your sensitive, loving care encourages them to explore the world. Over time, they learn they are separate from you and that when you leave, you always come back. With support, your baby will feel safe enough to trust another caring adult.

2

Visualize yourself accompanying your baby to the daycare or childcare provider during their settling-in period, staying with them initially.

3

Imagine their first full day in childcare. Picture you and your baby enjoying cuddles that morning. When you leave, your goodbye is short and sweet. Your baby will sense your confidence in leaving them—easing their anxiety. You understand that this feels sad (for both of you). Afterward, visualize how you may feel—letting yourself cry and soothing yourself.

4

Visualize the reunion with your baby and snuggling them. Reflect on the benefits of this change for you and for your baby—giving you time to reconnect to other identities, so important for your sense of self.

5

Practice other separations. Whenever you leave your baby, however briefly, say goodbye and remind them that you're coming back.

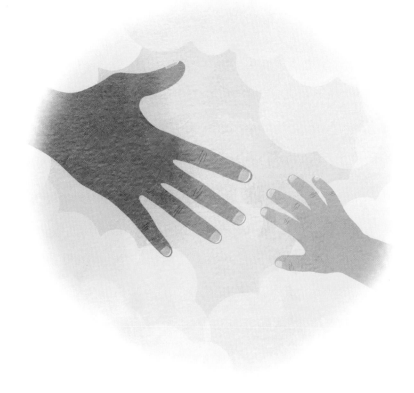

Coping with Emotions

As your baby turns one and begins to blossom into a spirited toddler, support them to explore the world with curiosity and delight. As they strive for independence, a common challenge is mindfully managing meltdowns.

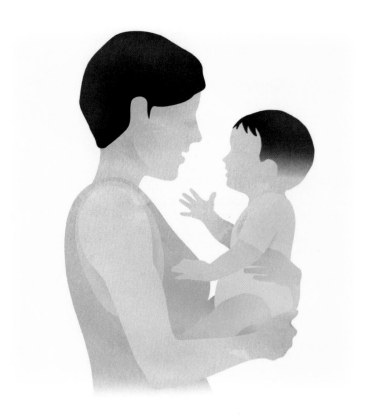

1

Reflect on how far you have come with your baby—now an active explorer who loves adventures with you. But how will you respond when they become a screaming bundle of emotions?

2

Witnessing your child upset may trigger strong emotions in you and fears of external judgment, such as: "What must other parents think?" or "I can't handle this."

3

Use your breath to calm yourself first and shrink down fear-based beliefs. Breathe deeply— breathe in for three counts, breathe out for six.

4

Imagine yourself, steady as an oak tree, rooted with your baby. Remember that other parents aren't judging you—they're thinking, "Poor you. I've been there, too!"

5

After self-soothing, focus on your child. Acknowledge, name, and validate their big feelings. Come down to their level and reassure them.

6

Remember that sometimes you have to hold a boundary and just sit with their distress and your own discomfort.

7

Afterward, be gentle with yourself. Reset through meditation, music, or calling a friend. Give yourself grace. It's not easy, but you're equipping your child to understand their rich emotions. And you're learning so much about your own emotions. Feel proud.

Practice and Posture

Yoga unites breath, body, and mind. Whether you reserve 10 or 30 minutes for gentle stretching and mental calm, allow your mind to observe your breath as you restore, release, and reenergize.

Mothering can leave us feeling "touched out," squeezed of physical and mental space. You may feel like your to-do list is never quite complete—if only you could check everything off. Yoga is a powerful reminder to focus on your journey rather than the destination. Notice your breath as it comes and goes, bringing your attention to your body. Giving yourself time to pause allows you to listen to what's going on internally. What feelings and sensations are you aware of? Take up an Observer position ... and simply notice.

"Carve out time for yourself, reminding yourself of the mantra: I am worthy of this space."

30-MINUTE SEQUENCE

Continue to listen to your body, be gentle with yourself, and transition carefully between each pose. If you wish, use aids to enhance relaxation, such as burning a scented candle and playing ambient music.

01

DYNAMIC CHILD'S POSE

From kneeling, softly allow your upper body to fold forward over your thighs. Rest your head on a block. Stretch your arms out in front of you, shoulder-width apart. Breathe comfortably, extend your arms, and draw your tailbone back. On each exhale, imagine stretching in both directions. Hold for as long as feels comfortable.

Draw your hips backward to stretch your body

Draw your shoulder blades away from each other

Extend along your arms and out through your hands

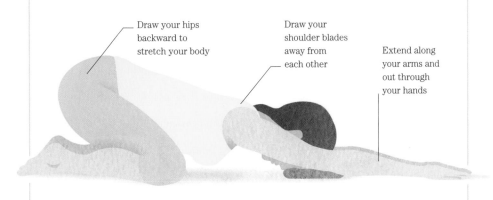

02

ONE-LEGGED PLANK

This is a gentle way to start engaging your core muscles.
Come into Tabletop, knees apart, hands aligned under your
shoulders. Press your hands into the floor and softly engage
your pelvic floor. Stretch one leg back and tuck your toes
under. Breathe in, and, as you breathe out, hold your pelvis
steady and push through your back heel. Bring your
attention to your breath, engage your pelvic floor softly,
and hold for a couple of breaths. Return to Tabletop, then
repeat with the other leg. When comfortable, progress to
a full plank, extending one leg back and then the other.

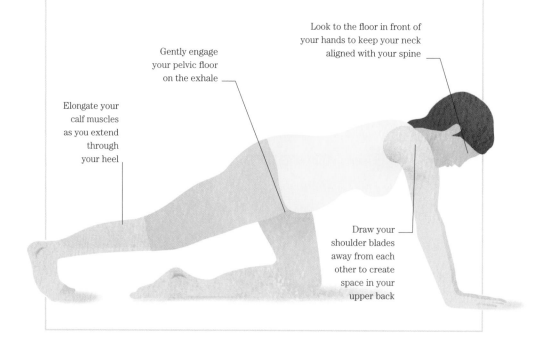

Look to the floor in front of
your hands to keep your neck
aligned with your spine

Gently engage
your pelvic floor
on the exhale

Elongate your
calf muscles
as you extend
through
your heel

Draw your
shoulder blades
away from each
other to create
space in your
upper back

03

PRESS-UP FROM KNEES

This exercise focuses on upper body and core strength, which will help with carrying your baby. From Tabletop, softly draw your body forward, bringing your shoulders slightly past your wrists. Bend your elbows and begin lowering your chest down toward the space between your hands, but go down only as far as feels comfortable. At first, you may move only a little way down. Hold briefly, then hug your belly toward your lower back and push up to straighten your arms and return to Tabletop. Repeat three to five times, as comfortable.

ENGAGE YOUR BABY

If you wish, position your baby near you so they can watch you and you can kiss them before you push up.

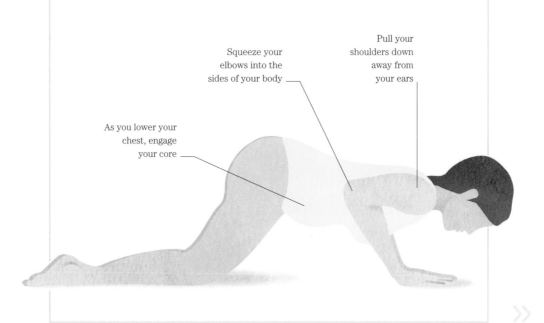

Squeeze your elbows into the sides of your body

Pull your shoulders down away from your ears

As you lower your chest, engage your core

04

SPHINX

Lie down flat on your stomach and extend your legs back, keeping them straight and on the floor. Bring your elbows directly under your shoulders and reach your forearms forward on the floor in front of you. Lift your chest and head up. Breathe comfortably. On the exhale, gently engage your pelvic floor muscles. Ground your pelvis and the tops of your feet down into the floor as you draw the heart area forward. Hold for up to 1 minute if comfortable. Repeat up to three times.

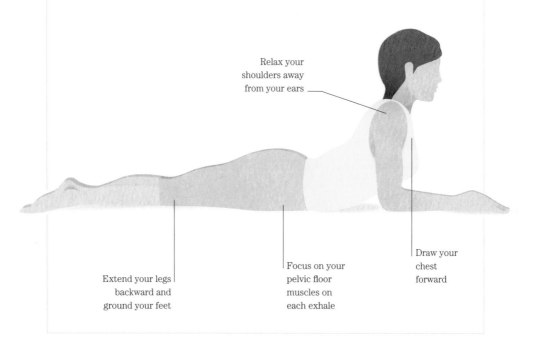

Relax your shoulders away from your ears

Draw your chest forward

Focus on your pelvic floor muscles on each exhale

Extend your legs backward and ground your feet

05

ELBOW PLANK

From Sphinx, interlace your fingers and lift your gaze toward your hands. Tuck your toes under and softly engage your pelvic floor and belly. If comfortable, draw back through your heels, allowing your belly, pelvis, and thighs to lift off the ground, remaining parallel to the floor. Breathe comfortably for 3–5 breaths. When ready, lower your hips down and rest in Sphinx. Repeat two to three times, then carefully stand up.

ADVANCED EXERCISE

Do this elbow plank only if you can comfortably breathe while holding this pose.

Hold your pelvis steady and engage your pelvic floor

Lengthen along your spine in both directions

Keep your shoulders down away from your ears

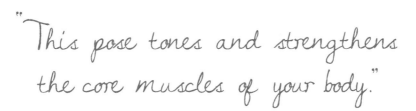

"This pose tones and strengthens the core muscles of your body."

06

TREE POSE

Stand in Mountain Pose and find a point of focus in front of you for stability. Let your weight rock onto your right foot and then externally rotate your left leg, allowing your knee to open outward. Bring your left foot to rest on the inner part of your right leg. Ground into your supporting leg. Engage your pelvic floor and extend your arms up to the sky. Breathe comfortably and hold for as long as comfortable, then repeat on the other side.

Reach upward from your waist

Softly engage your pelvic floor for stability

Rest your foot where it feels comfortable

Ground into your supporting leg

07

WARRIOR POSE

From Mountain Pose, glide your right foot back as far as possible while maintaining your balance. Bend your left knee toward the space over your left ankle. Keep your pelvis square, extend your right foot through your heel, and engage your right buttock for stability. Raise your arms up to the sky. Breathe comfortably for 5 breaths, then reach your arms forward and use the strength of your front leg to bring your back leg forward. Repeat on the other side.

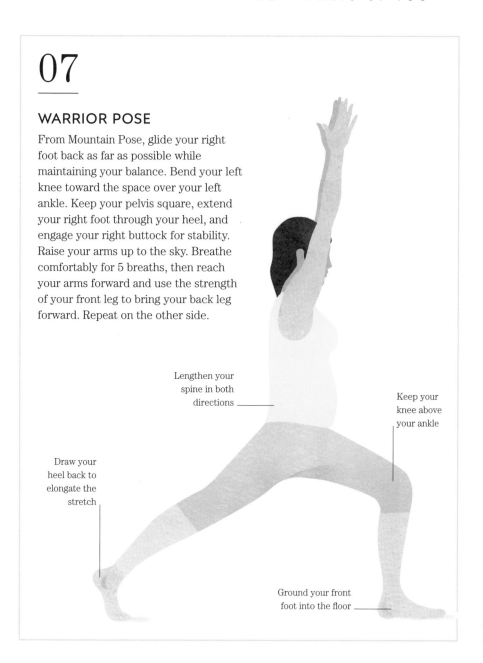

Lengthen your spine in both directions

Keep your knee above your ankle

Draw your heel back to elongate the stretch

Ground your front foot into the floor

08

LYING DOWN TWIST

Lie on your back and draw your knees up to your chest. Softly rock from side to side, enjoying a gentle massage of your lower back. When ready, allow both knees to drop over to the right, drawing them in toward your chest and resting your right arm on your knee. Breathe comfortably and allow your left arm to reach out to the side and diagonally upward for a stretch along the front of your chest and under arm. Allow your head to rest comfortably, turning to face the same direction as your extended arm if you wish. Hold for 5–10 breaths. Repeat on the other side.

Reach your arm out and diagonally upward

Let your breath flow naturally

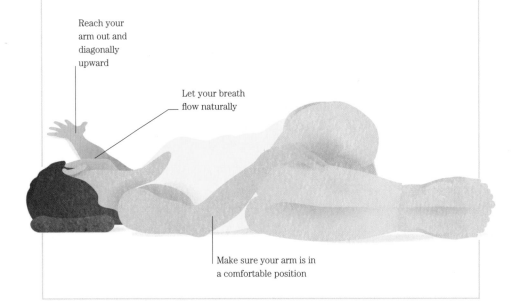

Make sure your arm is in a comfortable position

09

RESTORATIVE POSE

Place a few stacked pillows (or a bolster) on the floor and sit with your lower back against the short end of the pillows. Slowly lie your back along the length of the pillows, using your arms to aid you, so your back feels supported and comfortable. Add extra support under your head if needed. Once settled, let your arms relax out to the side and your legs extend outward. Breathe comfortably and enjoy this restful pose for up to 15 minutes or as long as feels comfortable.

Keep your neck long

Don't let your lower back overarch

Relax your legs

Let your arms gently settle onto the floor

"Pause to rest. With each exhale, soften, release, and let go."

WHERE TO SEEK HELP

Don't delay reaching out for help as things can spiral quickly. For emergency help, visit your local emergency department or urgent care; call 911; or make an urgent OB appointment.

Pre- and postnatal support

BabyCenter Community
community.babycenter.com

The New Parent Support Program
(for military families)
militaryonesource.mil/family-relationships/
parenting-and-children/parenting-infants-and-
toddlers/the-new-parent-support-program

American Baby Magazine
parents.com/american-baby-magazine

Mental Health America: Maternal Mental
Health
mhanational.org/maternal-mental-health

Substance Abuse and Mental Health Services
Administration (SAMHSA)
samhsa.gov/find-help/national-helpline

Birth trauma support

Postpartum Support International
postpartum.net

Make Birth Better
www.makebirthbetter.org

Psychological support

If any of this book's content triggers strong emotions, please talk to someone supportive. If you are struggling emotionally, your doctor can refer you to a local psychology service if appropriate and advise you on local self-help groups and mental health organizations offering support.

If you have the means and wish to access private talking therapy, you could start by visiting the Psychology Today: Find a Therapist (psychologytoday.com/us/therapists) or TalkSpace (talkspace.com).

Action on Postpartum Psychosis
www.app-network.org

American College of Obstetricians and
Gynecologists: Postpartum Depression
acog.org/womens-health/faqs/postpartum-
depression

www.drcarolineboyd.com/infant-related-harm-
thoughts (unwanted intrusive thoughts)

American Psychiatric Association
psychiatry.org/patients-families

March of Dimes: Stillbirth
www.marchofdimes.org/complications/
stillbirth.aspx

Breastfeeding support

www.kellymom.com

La Leche League
lllusa.org

WIC Breastfeeding Support (USDA)
wicbreastfeeding.fns.usda.gov

USEFUL RESOURCES

Baby massage and yoga

International Association of Infant Massage
iaim.net

Yoga babies
www.yogababies.co.uk

Yoga nidra
www.yoganidranetwork.org

Compassion and mindfulness

Calm; Clementine; Headspace (apps)

www.compassionatemind.co.uk

www.coherentbreathing.org

www.self-compassion.org

www.tarabrach.com/guided-meditations

Containment and reciprocity

www.solihullapproachparenting.com

Recommended reading

M. Cree, *The Compassionate Mind Approach to Postnatal Depression: Using Compassion Focused Therapy to Enhance Mood, Confidence and Bonding*, Robinson (2015).

P. Gilbert, *The Compassionate Mind*, Robinson (2009).

J. Kabat-Zinn and M. Kabat-Zinn, *Everyday Blessings: Mindfulness for Parents*, Piatkus (2014).

REFERENCES

General

N. Bardacke, *Mindful Birthing: Training the Mind, Body, and Heart for Childbirth and Beyond*, HarperCollins (2012).

M. Cree, *The Compassionate Mind Approach to Postnatal Depression: Using Compassion Focused Therapy to Enhance Mood, Confidence and Bonding*, Robinson (2015).

P. Gilbert, *The Compassionate Mind*, Robinson (2009).

R. Harris, *The Happiness Trap: Stop Struggling, Start Living*, Robinson (2011).

J. Kabat-Zinn and M. Kabat-Zinn, *Everyday Blessings: Mindfulness for Parents*, Piatkus (2014).

A. Mathur, *Mind Over Mother*, Piatkus (2020).

P. Nicolson, *Postnatal Depression: Facing the Paradox of Loss, Happiness and Motherhood*, Wiley-Blackwell (2001).

O. Serrallach, *The Postnatal Depletion Cure: A Complete Guide to Rebuilding Your Health and Reclaiming Your Energy for Mothers of Newborns, Toddlers and Young Children*, Sphere (2018).

N. Stadlen, *What Mothers Do: Especially When It Looks Like Nothing*, Piatkus (2004).

J. Ussher, *Managing the Monstrous Feminine: Regulating the Reproductive Body*, Routledge (2006).

K. Whittingham, *Becoming Mum*, Pivotal Publishing (2015).

NHS, "The Solihull Approach," NHS Solihull Approach [web page], www.solihullapproachparenting.com (accessed May–Aug 2021).

Page 10
J. Kabat-Zinn, "Mindfulness-based Interventions in Context: Past, Present, and Future," *Clinical Psychology: Science and Practice* 10, no. 2 (2003), pp144–156.

Page 12
E. S. Potharst et al., "Mindful With Your Baby: Feasibility, Acceptability, and Effects of a Mindful Parenting Group Training for Mothers and Their Babies in a Mental Health Context," *Mindfulness* 8 (2017), pp1236–1250.

C. C. Turpyn et al., "Affective Neural Mechanisms of a Parenting-focused Mindfulness Intervention," *Mindfulness* 12 (2021), pp392–404.

Page 14
E. Hoekzema et al., "Pregnancy Leads to Long-lasting Changes in Human Brain Structure," *Nature Neuroscience* 20 (2017), pp287–296.

D. Raphael, "Matrescence, Becoming a Mother, A 'New/Old' Rite de Passage," *Being Female*, De Gruyter Mouton (2011), pp65–72.

A. Sacks, "A New Way to Think about the Transition to Motherhood," TED [web video], May 2018, www.ted.com/talks/alexandra_sacks_a_new_way_to_think_about_the_transition_to_motherhood.

Page 16
P. Choi et al., "Supermum, Superwife, Supereverything: Performing Femininity in the Transition to Motherhood," *Journal of Reproductive and Infant Psychology* 23, no. 2 (2005), pp167–180.

K. Russell et al., *Maternal Mental Health—Women's Voices*, Royal College of Obstetricians and Gynaecologists (2017).

Pages 17 and 113
D. W. Winnicott, *Playing and Reality*, Tavistock Publications (1971).

Pages 20–21
P. Fonagy and E. Allison, "What is Mentalization? The Concept and its Foundations in Developmental Research," *Minding the Child*, Routledge (2013), pp25–48.

Three Circle model adapted from P. Gilbert, *The Compassionate Mind*, Robinson (2009). With permission from Little, Brown Book Group Ltd.

P. Gilbert, "The Origins and Nature of Compassion Focused Therapy," *British Journal of Clinical Psychology* 53, no.1 (2014), pp6–41.

Page 23
K. Le Nguyen et al., "Loving-kindness Meditation Slows Biological Aging in Novices: Evidence from a 12-week Randomized Controlled Trial," *Psychoneuroendocrinology* 108 (2019), pp20–27.

Pages 23 and 27
B. Hölzel et al., "Mindfulness Practice Leads to Increases in Regional Brain Gray Matter Density," *Psychiatry Research: Neuroimaging* 191, no. 1 (2011), pp36–43.

Page 27
M. J. Schroevers et al., "Is Learning Mindfulness Associated with Improved Affect

After Mindfulness-based Cognitive Therapy?" *British Journal of Psychology* 101, no. 1 (2010), pp95–107.

M. Williams et al., *Mindfulness: A Practical Guide to Finding Peace in a Frantic World*, Piatkus (2011).

Page 33
B. Knechtle et al., "Cold Water Swimming-Benefits and Risks: A Narrative Review," *International Journal of Environmental Research and Public Health* 17, no. 23 (2020).

Page 34
R. Bragg et al., "Ecominds: Effects on Mental Wellbeing," *Mind* (2013), pp1–112.

A. McGeeney, *With Nature in Mind: The Ecotherapy Manual for Mental Health Professionals*, Jessica Kingsley Publishers (2016).

Page 35
T. Field, "Infant Massage Therapy Research Review," *Clinical Research in Pediatrics* 1, no. 2 (2018), pp1–9.

Pages 36–9
C. L. Dennis et al., "Traditional Postpartum Practices and Rituals: A Qualitative Systematic Review," *Women's Health* 3, no. 4 (2007), pp487–502.

Page 44
K. M. Robson and R. Kumar, "Delayed Onset of Maternal Affection after Childbirth," *The British Journal of Psychiatry* 136, no. 4 (1980), pp347–353.

Page 46
W. Hollway, "Rereading Winnicott's 'Primary Maternal Preoccupation,'" *Feminism and Psychology* 22, no. 1 (2012), pp20–40.

Page 67
R. E. Moore et al., "Early Skin-to-skin Contact for Mothers and their Healthy Newborn Infants," *Cochrane Database of Systematic Reviews* 11 (2016).

Page 68
D. Daws, "A Child Psychotherapist in the Baby Clinic of a General Practice," *Reflecting on Reality: Psychotherapists at Work in Primary Care*, Routledge (2005), pp18–36.

Page 71
NICE, "Antenatal and Postnatal Mental Health: Clinical Management and Service guidance" NICE Guidance [web page], Guidance 1 Recommendations (2014), www.nice.org.uk/guidance/cg192/chapter/1-recommendations (accessed May–Aug 2021).

Page 110
N. K. Law et al., "Common Negative Thoughts in Early Motherhood and Their Relationship to Guilt, Shame and Depression," *Journal of Child and Family Studies* 30 (2021), pp1–15.

Page 113
E. Z. Tronick, "Emotions and Emotional Communication in Infants," *American Psychologist* 44, no. 2 (1989), pp112–119.

Page 125
N. Jones, "Babies' Musical Memories Formed in Womb," *New Scientist* [web article], July 2001, www.newscientist.com/article/dn994-babies-musical-memories-formed-in-womb (accessed May–Aug 2021).

Pages 136–37
Exercise adapted from K. Whittingham, *Becoming Mum*, Pivotal Publishing (2015).

Page 149
C. Boyd and K. Gannon, "How Do New/recent Mothers Experience Unwanted Thoughts of Harm Related to their Newborn? A Thematic Analysis," *Journal of Reproductive and Infant Psychology* 37, no. 5 (2019).

N. Fairbrother, "Perinatal Obsessive-compulsive Disorder and Infant-related Harm Thoughts: Prevalence and Relation to Infant Safety." Academic Perinatology Rounds, BC Women's Hospital and Health Centre, Vancouver, BC; Presenter. June 2021.

Page 151
S. Fraiberg et al., "Ghosts in the Nursery:
A Psychoanalytic Approach to the Problems
of Impaired Infant-mother Relationships,"
*Journal of the American Academy of Child
Psychiatry* 14, no. 3 (1975), pp387–422.

Page 160
B. Elliott, "The 9 Best Foods and Drinks to
Have Before Bed," *Healthline* [web article],
August 2020, www.healthline.com/nutrition/9-
foods-to-help-you-sleep (accessed May–Aug
2021).

Pages 162–3
Exercise adapted from R. Harris, *ACT Made
Simple*, New Harbinger Publications, Inc.
(2009); and S. Hayes and S. Smith, *Get Out of
Your Mind and into Your Life*, New
Harbinger Publications, Inc. (2005).

Page 165
S. M. Chang et al., "Effects of an Intervention
with Drinking Chamomile Tea on Sleep Quality
and Depression in Sleep Disturbed Postnatal
Women: A Randomized Controlled Trial,"
Journal of Advanced Nursing 72, no. 2
(2016), pp306–315.

Page 173
Exercise adapted from T. Brach, "RAIN:
Recognize, Allow, Investigate, Nurture,"
T. Brach [web page], www.tarabrach.com/rain
(accessed May–Aug 2021).

Pages 187 and 189
A. Daminger, "The Cognitive Dimension of
Household Labor," *American Sociological
Review* 84, no. 4 (2019), pp609–633.

A. McMunn et al., "Gender Divisions of Paid
and Unpaid Work in Contemporary UK
Couples," *Work, Employment and Society* 34,
no. 2 (2019), pp155–173.

Page 191
G. J. Privitera et al., "Proximity and Visibility of
Fruits and Vegetables Influence Intake in a
Kitchen Setting Among College Students,"
Environment and Behavior (2012).

Page 195
The Gottman Institute [web page] www.
gottman.com (accessed May–Aug 2021).

Page 198
E. Rodsky, *Fair Play: A Game-changing
Solution for When You Have Too Much to
Do (and More Life to Live)*, Quercus (2019).

To access the complete list of source materials,
studies, and research supporting the text in
this book, visit: www.dk.com/mnm-biblio

Index

ACKNOWLEDGMENTS

From the Author

Giving birth to this baby has been an honor, requiring me to recenter myself each day (sometimes, each hour). I've tried to stay mindful along the way—imperfectly, of course! With loving thanks to Laurie, my husband, my shipmate, my patient proofreader. To my two children, Isla and Reuben, whose existence prompted my doctoral research and, now, this book. Your love and spirit grounds me each day. Thank you also to my parents and in-laws, for your encouragement and kindness, and my late father, who first introduced me to meditation 25 years ago.

Just as it takes a village to raise a child, it takes one to write a book about mothering, too. Thank you to Claire Wedderburn-Maxwell for your warm and thoughtful editorial guidance, and to Dawn Henderson for believing in me. To the DK team for working so hard to make such a beautiful book that I hope will reassure and anchor new moms. To my lovely supervisor, Dr. Sara Anderson, for your wisdom, feedback, and containing presence (as always). To my wonderful yoga teacher, Sunnah Rose, for generously giving your time and expertise.

My heartfelt thanks to my therapist, AG, and Drs. Faye Nikopaschos, Nicola Jacyna, Sarah Rowe, and Helen Sharples for your wise counsel and support, and to Sharon Lee Plaskitt and Dr. Rebecca Moore for your invaluable suggestions and guidance. A huge thank you to Jay Ehrlich; registered dietician Nichola Ludlam-Raine; Anya Hayes, author of *The Supermum Myth* and *Postnatal Pilates*; massage therapist Hannah Johnson; nutritionist Thalia Pellegrini; and yoga nidra teacher Sara Johnson, for sharing your wisdom, insights, and expertise. Sincere thanks to Mothers At Home Matter, Dr. Tina Mistry, and Kemi Omijeh for helping with recruitment, and to the mothers who share their experiences powerfully in this book. And finally, thank you to my clients and the moms who speak to me on Instagram for your courage and spirit and from whom I learn so much. Let's keep taking action to increase compassion for all mothers.

From the Publisher

DK would like to thank Jane Ellis for proofreading and Hilary Bird for indexing.

DISCLAIMER

Every effort has been made to ensure that the information in this book is complete and accurate. However, neither the publisher nor the author is engaged in rendering professional advice or services to the individual reader. The ideas, advice, and suggestions contained in this book are not intended as a substitute for consulting with your health-care provider. All matters regarding the health of you and your baby require medical supervision. Consult with your health-care provider before undertaking any of the aromatherapy, nutrition, exercises, techniques, natural remedies, and alternative therapies set out in this book. Neither the author nor the publisher shall be liable or responsible for any loss or damage allegedly arising from any information or suggestion in this book.

ABOUT THE AUTHOR

Clinical psychologist **Dr. Caroline Boyd** has an MA in classics, an MSc in psychology, and a doctorate in clinical psychology. She has more than 10 years' experience working in the National Health Service in the UK and mental health settings and specializes in supporting new parents in her independent psychology practice, Parent Therapy Hub.

Caroline works with parents around all aspects of the transition—from pregnancy to childbirth and beyond. She adopts a holistic approach to well-being, and her published research explores mothers' experiences of intrusive thoughts about their babies. Caroline speaks at conferences, including the annual Birth Trauma conference, and shares psychology ideas on Instagram, her blog, and podcasts such as *Motherkind* to help parents feel more connected—to themselves and their children—and less alone.

You can follow Caroline on Instagram @_drboyd

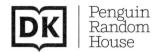

Project Editor Claire Wedderburn-Maxwell
Project Designer Vanessa Hamilton
Senior Designer Barbara Zuniga
Senior Editor Dawn Titmus
Editor Kiron Gill
US Editor Jennette ElNaggar
Editorial Assistant Charlotte Beauchamp
Jacket Coordinator Lucy Philpott
Jacket Designer Amy Cox
Senior Production Editor Tony Phipps
Senior Production Controller Luca Bazzoli
Creative Technical Support Sonia Charbonnier
Managing Editor Dawn Henderson
Design Manager Marianne Markham
Art Director Maxine Pedliham
Publishing Director Katie Cowan

Illustrator Keith Hagan
Photographer Ruth Jenkinson
Prop Stylist Robert Merrett
Food Stylist Isabel de Cordova

First American Edition, 2022
Published in the United States by DK Publishing
1450 Broadway, Suite 801, New York, NY 10018

Text copyright © Dr. Caroline Boyd
Copyright © 2022 Dorling Kindersley Limited
DK, a Division of Penguin Random House LLC
22 23 24 25 26 10 9 8 7 6 5 4 3 2 1
001–326295–March/2022

A catalog record for this book
is available from the Library of Congress.
ISBN 978-0-7440-5348-7

Printed and bound in China

For the curious
www.dk.com

This book was made with Forest
Stewardship Council™ certified paper—
one small step in DK's commitment to a
sustainable future. For more information
go to www.dk.com/our-green-pledge